e.a.t.

A Journal for What You Eat, and for What's Eating You!

written & created by Forbes Riley

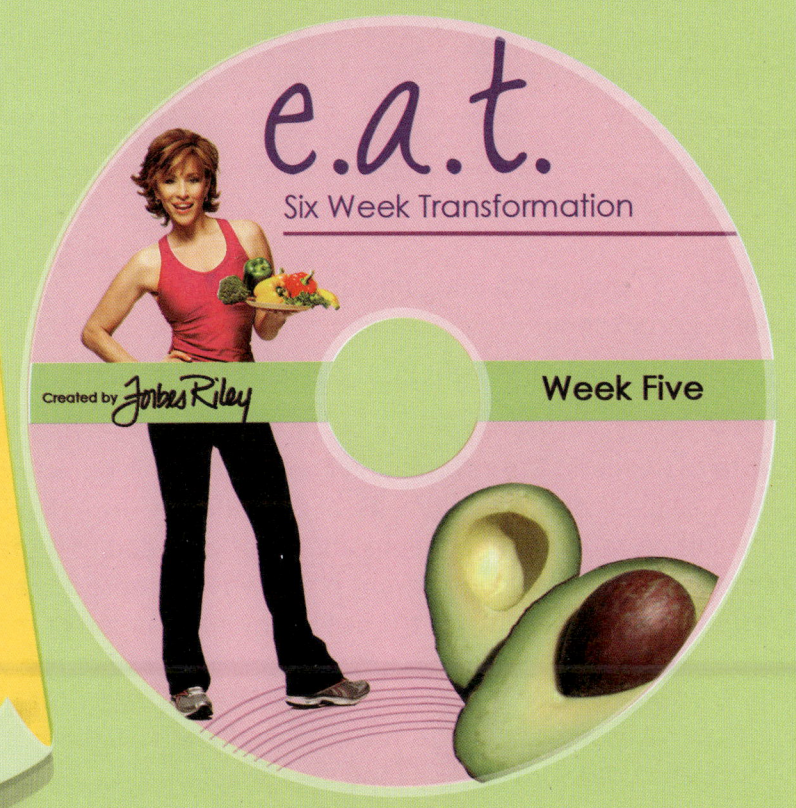

congratulations!

The first step is to watch the "Get Started" video.

www.MyeatJournal.com

Let's do this together!

e.a.t.
Six Week Transformation

Created by Forbes Riley

Week Five

All right reserved. No part of this book may be reproduced or transmitted in any form or by any means, electronic or mechanical, including photocopying, recording, or by any information storage and retrieval system, with permission in writing from the publisher.

Copyright c 2013 by Forbes Riley & Midvale Direct LLC

Published by Midvale Direct LLC, Los Angeles, CA

Visit us on the web!
www.myeatjournal.com
www.fitwithforbes.com
facebook: https://facebook.com/forbesrileyFANpage

E-mail us at: info@EatJournal.com

Printed in the United States of America

Written & Created by Forbes Riley, Graphic Design by Jaki Hale

ISBN 78-0-9888747-0-1

First Edition

Library of Congress Cataloging-in-Publication Data
Riley, Forbes 1960-
1. Eating Journal 2. Weight loss 3. Health 4. Nutrition 5. Mind & Body

Note to Readers: The information contained in this book, including nutritional advice, diet plans, exercise plans or other regimens, and all other information is the result of experience and research by the author, reflects her opinions and is not intended to replace medical advice. Before beginning any diet or exercise plan consult your physician to be sure it is appropriate for you. The author accepts no responsibility or liability for the use of any information or material contained in this book.

> *This book is dedicated to all the people who struggle in the dark* with their weight and feel "less than" - I have been where you are and there is a light at the end of the tunnel. There is a way to live everyday with joy, eat food, be sociable and fit in – no matter what size you are.
>
> I especially dedicate this journal to my Mom.
> So beautiful on the inside and out - she fought her own personal body image struggle throughout her life and mine. May she rest in peace with the knowledge that I am committed to helping others live with freedom, joy and passion about themselves.

FORBES Riley

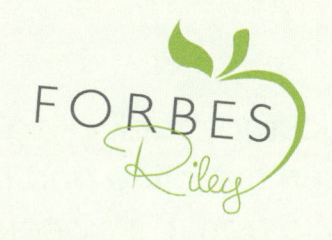

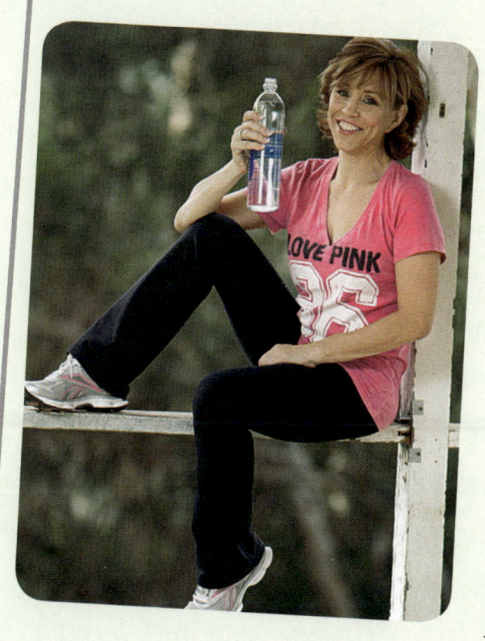

Dear Friend,

I am so excited to share this journal with you. To me it represents the rainbow at the end of a tunnel filled with struggle, heartache and frustration over food, my weight and my personal image. It's an honor to offer up this book as inspiration to help you with your transformation. I know it works! It worked for me and for countless other people who have chosen to commit to positive change in their lives.

I like to eat, no scratch that, I LOVE to eat! Holidays, celebrations, parties... even depression, all have food associations with them. Now, thanks to journaling, getting educated about food and being honest with myself, I don't live to eat... I eat to live.

To e.a.t. does not mean to stuff your face, to squash down feelings, or to stand in front of the refrigerator late at night binging. To e.a.t. does not mean finishing everything on your plate, downing an entire bag of chips or even counting calories . . . so, let's redefine e.a.t. once and for all!

e.a.t. = Enjoying All Tastes

Wow! if that's what e.a.t. means, THEN, it might mean enjoying a taste for all food, enjoying a taste for life, a taste for love, excitement and a taste for all the success that life has to offer.

And you thought this was just a food diary. Think again! My unique journal is chock-full of tips and inspiration along with motivating, thought provoking exercises. Ultimately when you complete this journey, you'll have made new habits and you'll never feel compelled to go on someone else's diet again... you'll have created your own!

Shall we get started?

Sincerely, *Forbes Riley*

Why Journal?

I started writing in a daily journal back in high school as part of a creative writing class and have been exploring and tinkering with the process throughout my life. I have to admit, it's been fun and enlightening to go back through my old journals and relive what I was experiencing and thinking during various times in my life. Sadly, though, most of my journals started with my frustration about being overweight and a new commitment to losing those unwanted pounds. I must have written about it a hundred different times, recorded every diet I ever tried, counted all the calories I consumed and every success and failure I endured. The process of writing down food began to make me conscious of what I was eating - I often think back to when I mindlessly devoured a whole bag of potato chips, an entire carton of chocolate chip cookies, or heaven forbid someone left a container of ice cream in the freezer. I was under the illusion that I was eating healthy (*ice cream has milk in it, doesn't it?*) but I simply couldn't figure out why I was always 25-35 lbs overweight. Turns out, food was only one part of my issue; it wasn't until my 30's that I began to realize the underlying problems weren't necessarily WHAT I was eating, but WHY I was eating. Those explorations finally lead to my deep understanding of how I used food as an excuse and escape and ultimately helped me come to grips with my eating compulsions.

So why is THIS journal different?

I created e.a.t. because I found most journals were poorly designed or blank books with no plan, lacking motivation and with no end in sight. e.a.t. is unique because it's designed to be a 6 week non-diet commitment, chock-full of motivation, landmarks and hints along the way to keep you on target. It contains daily exercises and affirmations to help in the systematic release of some of the issues we keep bottled up (*and maybe don't even realize*) that are affecting our daily eating habits.

According to Kaiser Permanente's Center for Healthy Research - "keeping a daily food diary can help increase a patients weight loss. It seems the simple act of writing down what you eat can encourage you to consume fewer calories, monitor your eating habits and provide insight for your doctor."

Do you eat when you are frustrated, angry, depressed?

Emotional issues behind overeating are often the biggest obstacle for many of us. Indulging and out of control behavior often causes us to beat ourselves up - it literally **eats** at us and often we just feel helpless. Writing about these feelings can help liberate them.

Another key to successful weight loss is understanding WHAT you are eating; the affect that sugar has on your body, controlling portion size and consuming enough nutrition for successful bodily function... but this awareness doesn't happen overnight. It's a process and an education. You didn't get to this weight or emotional state overnight.

Together let us embark on this 6-week adventure with an open mind, a ready heart and a belief in you. Your commitment contract is below, fill in your name (twice), sign, date it and ...

let's get started!

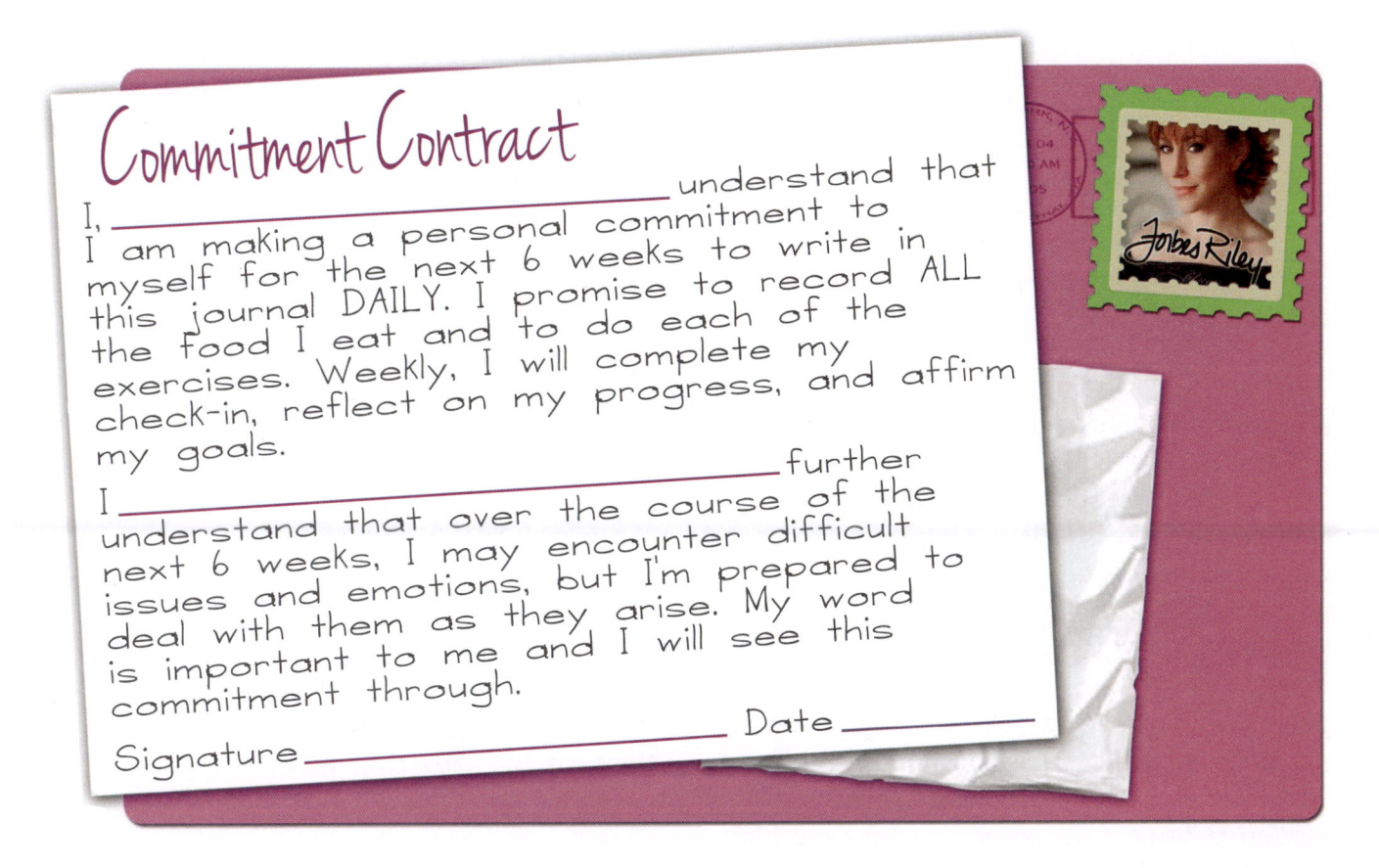

Commitment Contract

I, _____ understand that I am making a personal commitment to myself for the next 6 weeks to write in this journal DAILY. I promise to record ALL the food I eat and to do each of the exercises. Weekly, I will complete my check-in, reflect on my progress, and affirm my goals.

I _____ further understand that over the course of the next 6 weeks, I may encounter difficult issues and emotions, but I'm prepared to deal with them as they arise. My word is important to me and I will see this commitment through.

Signature _____ Date _____

First Thing You Need to Do
Clean Out & Restock Your Kitchen!

Essentials

Whole Grains: Brown rice, oatmeal, cream of wheat, quinoa, wasa crackers.

Nuts/Seeds: Raw unsalted almonds, cashews, sunflower seeds, chia seeds, organic peanut butter, sunflower seeds, almond butter.

Cereals: Kashi cereals, mueslis, bran flakes.

Dried Fruit: Apricots, dates, raisins, dried apples, prunes, cranberries, figs.

Condiments: Mustard, salsa, organic ketchup, honey, low calorie jelly/jam, vinegar (balsamic, apple cider, wine), herbs (parsley, thyme, oregano, sea salt, pepper, capers, basil, chive, fennel, dill, coriander, rosemary, sage), garlic powder, low-sodium, vegetable or chicken broth, onion powder.

Oils: Extra virgin olive oil, safflower oil, coconut oil

Produce: A rainbow mix of fruits and vegetables including apples, apricots, artichokes, asparagus, avocado, bananas, blackberries, blueberries, broccoli, cabbage, cantaloupe, carrots, celery, cherries, coconut, cucumber, edamame, eggplant, garlic, grapes, grapefruit, green beans, honeydew melon, kiwi, kale, lemons, lettuce (romaine, butter), limes, mangos, nectarines, onions, oranges, papaya, peach, pear, pineapples, plums, pomegranates, potatoes, pumpkin, radish, raspberries, strawberries, snap peas, spinach, squash tangerine, tomato, watermelon, yams, zucchini.

Dry Goods: Baking soda, whole-grain flours, baking powder, vanilla.

Pantry: Unsweetened applesauce, chickpeas, lentils, kidney beans, canned tomatoes crushed, whole and diced, tuna water packed, salmon water packed, low-fat soups, lemon juice, lime juice.

Freezer: Whole-grain breads, whole-grain wraps, chicken breasts, steak, pork tenderloin, fish (salmon, tilapia, cod), frozen berries, frozen vegetables.

Refrigerator: Low-fat soy/almond milk, skim milk, eggs, low fat string cheese, low fat cottage cheese, nitrite free range chicken/turkey breast, steak, fish, fresh squeezed orange juice/ grapefruit juice/ pomegranate, hummus, guacamole, greek yogurt, olives.

Spice It Up

Spices: Red Pepper flakes, cinnamon, nutmeg, cloves, allspice.

Herbs: parsley, thyme, oregano, sea salt, pepper, capers, basil, chive, fenel, dill, coriander, rosemary, basil other favorites

Trash Bags: Throw out all of the cakes, candies, cookies, etc!

Food for Thought

Although this is not a diet program, it does help if you follow a few simple guidelines;

Don't Skip Meals
Many busy people with kids, careers or hectic schedules tend to miss breakfast or skip meals altogether - and then wonder why they can't seem to lose those stubborn pounds. When you don't eat for 4 or more hours you tend to slow you metabolism down and even though you may be eating less food, you're not burning it efficiently. The strategy of skipping a meal and catching up later will backfire. So eat every 3 or so hours and write it down in this journal.

Make Smart Choices
Fiber-rich whole food and lean protein help to stabilize blood sugar levels and help keep you feeling fuller for hours. You can power up your metabolism with nuts and proteins as a snack, so when its time for your next meal you're not ravenous - How many times have you said, "I'm starving" and then proceed to use that as an excuse to eat anything in sight. Have an apple, low-fat yogurt, a piece of string cheese or a handful of raw almonds.

A Toast to Change!
Calories from alcohol add up quickly (a regular beer has 150 calories, martinis about 140 calories, vodka/tequila/whiskey average 80 and wine about 100 per glass). Alcohol also makes you have enough "fun" that you might indulge in fattening choices and it decreases your body's fat burning process while stressing out your liver. A good choice might be club soda with a twist of lemon or lime.

CUT OUT SOME CALORIES - easily!
- Don't eat the taco salad shell of your taco salad
- Use a small plate when going through a buffet - fill it only once
- Sushi is good, sashimi (no rice) is better and pass on the fried tempura
- Chicken breasts have less calories than the thighs and legs
- Having canned tuna? Try water packed and pass on the oil
- Try substituting veggie or turkey burger for hamburgers
- Order your fish, meat and chicken with added sauces on the side
- Always order your salad with dressing on the side
- Don't let the waiters SHOW you the dessert tray - its too tempting!
- Have an urge for french fries? - try baking them at home (not fried)

Watch Portion Sizes
At home its easy to judge portion sizes and weigh ingredients; a bit more difficult at restaurants, so a good rule of thumb is to always ask for a doggy bag BEFORE you start eating.
Some easy ways to "eyeball" portion sizes -
- meat & chicken = the size of your palm
- pasta = the size of a tennis ball
- potato or yam = a computer mouse
- cheese = 6 dice
- fish = a checkbook

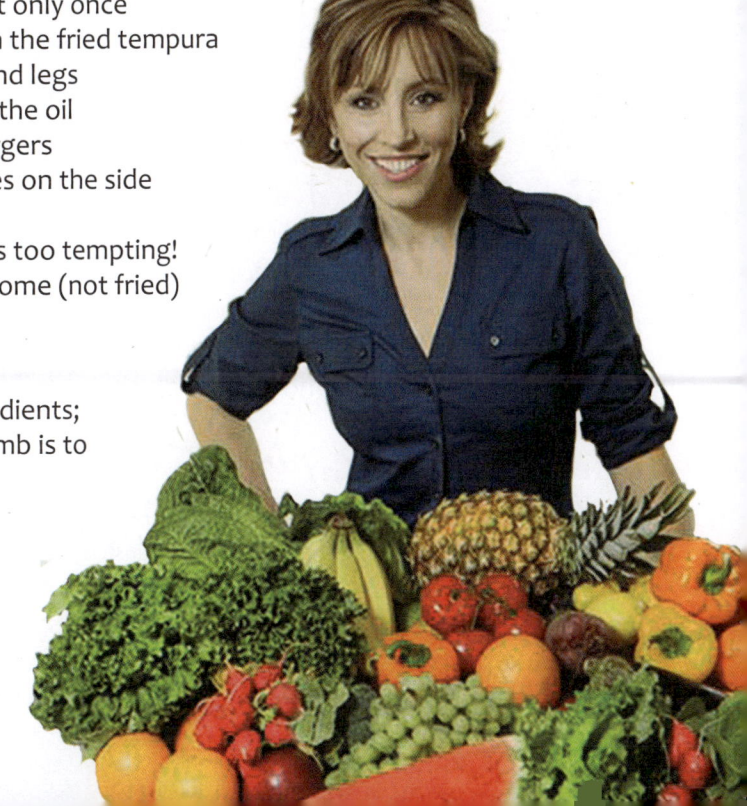

Quick & Healthy Meals

Breakfast
Under 300 calories

Quick & Out the Door
1 hard boiled egg
1 medium banana
12 raw almonds

The No Drive-Thru
Cook 1 egg in non-stick pan
Place egg, 1 slice cheddar cheese on a toasted whole-grain English muffin

4 Layer Perfect Parfait
Layer 4 oz nonfat vanilla Greek yogurt
Layer 2 tbsp. of chopped raw & unsalted nuts (walnuts, almonds, cashews)
1 cup berries (sliced strawberries, blueberries, raspberries)
Top with 4 oz nonfat vanilla Greek yogurt

Lunch
Under 350 calories

Home Delivery
Top 2 halves of a whole-wheat English muffin with 2 tsp low sugar tomato sauce, 1/4 cup shredded part skim mozzarella, broil until cheese melts and 1/2 sliced pear.

Soup & Sam
Heat 1-cup low-sodium tomato soup
Place 2 oz of low-sodium turkey breast (2 slices), tomato, lettuce, and 1 slice of low fat cheese, (swiss, cheddar) on 2 slices of whole grain bread.
Serve with a side of baby carrots

Burger Up!
Cook a 4 oz. turkey or veggie burger in a nonstick pan until done. Place on a whole-wheat bun; top with 1/2 tomato and 1/2 avocado, lettuce.

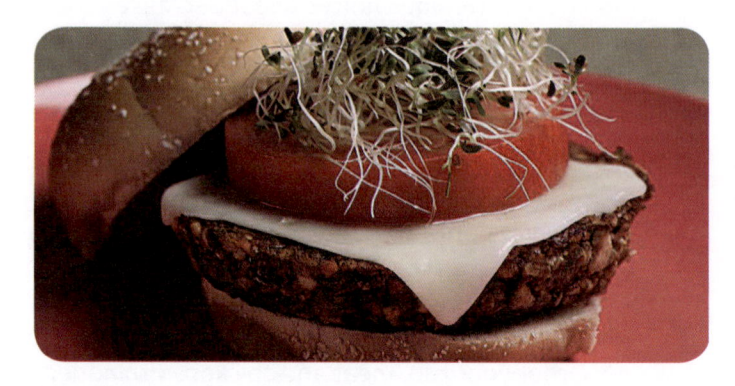

Dinner
Under 450 calories

Best Catch of the Day
In a glass bowl, prepare marinade by mixing 2 cloves minced garlic, 3 tsp olive oil, 1 tsp fresh basil, 1 tsp salt, 1 tbsp. lemon juice, and 1 tsp. fresh chopped parsley. Place 6 oz. salmon fillet in a glass baking dish and cover with marinade. Marinate in fridge for about 2 hours, turning occasionally. Preheat oven to 375 degrees. Place filet in aluminum foil, cover with marinate and seal. Place sealed salmon in the glass dish and bake for 35 to 45 minutes. Serve with side salad.

Homemade "Unfried" Chicken
Preheat oven to 375. In a shallow bowl combine 1/2 cup whole grain or panko breadcrumbs, 2 tbsp grated Parmesan, 2 tsp grated lemon zest, 1/2 tsp paprika, and a pinch of salt. In a second shallow bowl, mix 3 tbsp. fresh lemon juice, 1 tbsp water, and 1 tbsp olive oil. Coat a baking pan with cooking spray. Dip 4 boneless Chicken breasts (about 5 oz each) in a liquid mixture, then in breadcrumb mixture coating entire breast and lay on the baking pan. Bake 20 to 25 minutes until cooked through (no pink inside). Serve with steamed broccoli.

Creative Snacks
Under 400 calories

Wasabi Edamame
Cook 1 pound frozen edamame (green soybeans) according to package directions; drain. Immediately toss with 1 tablespoon fresh lime juice, 1 teaspoon wasabe paste and ¼ teaspoon salt.

Goat Cheese and Roasted Tomato Crostini
Preheat oven to 425 degrees. Combine 1 cup halved cherry tomatoes, 1 tablespoon olive oil, 1 sliced garlic clove, ¼ teaspoon salt, ½ teaspoon black pepper and ¼ cup fresh basil leaves; roast in middle of oven until tomatoes wilt and are golden (about 20 minutes). Remove from oven; drizzle with 2 teaspoons balsamic vinegar. Roast an additional 10 minutes. Spread ½ cup packaged herbed goat cheese evenly onto 12 toasted crostini; top with tomato mixture.

Oven Roasted Sweet Potato Chips
Preheat oven to 425 degrees. Cut sweet potatoes into ¼ inch-thick slices; set aside. Combine 1 tablespoon olive oil, 1 ½ teaspoons chili powder, ½ teaspoon salt and ¼ teaspoon ground cumin. Add sweet potatoes; toss gently to coat. Cover a lightly oiled non-stick baking sheet with a single layer of potatoes; roast, turning once, until golden and tender (about 20 minutes).

Fast Food Ideas (if you must!)
Under 400 calories

Breakfast
- McDonald's Egg McMuffin
- Panera Bread Pumpkin Muffin; kid-size organic yogurt
- Starbucks "Perfect Oatmeal" topped with chopped nuts
- Starbucks Egg White Turkey Bacon Breakfast

Lunch
- Arby's Ham and Swiss Melt Sandwich; applesauce
- Burger King Veggie Burger (hold the mayonnaise!)
- Subway 6-inch Oven Roasted Chicken Breast Sub; 1 bowl minestrone
- Wendy's Mandarin Chicken Salad w/ roasted almonds (use 1/2 packet of Oriental Sesame Dressing)
- Taco Bell chicken Burrito Supreme

Dinner
- Chik-Fil-A/ Burger King/ KFC - Grilled Chicken Sandwich
- Olive Garden- Herbed Grilled Salmon
- Pizza Hut- 2 slices Fit'n Delicious Diced Red Tomato, Mushroom Pizza
- Chipotle- 3 Steak Tacos (soft taco shells, steak, fajita vegetables, tomato salsa, lettuce)

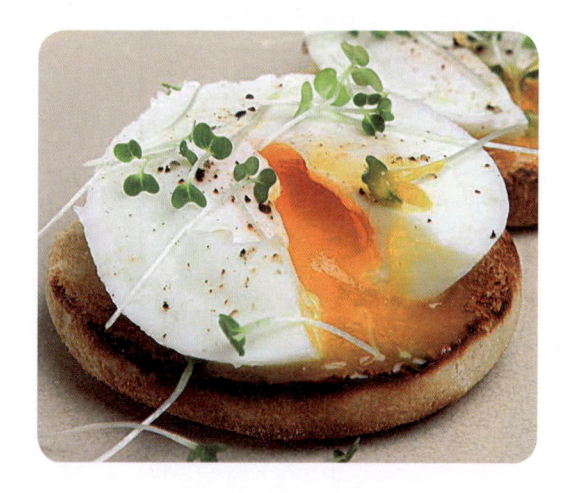

Food Labels - What DO you eat?

Serving Size: The first place to start when you look at a nutritional label is the serving size and the number of servings in the package. How many servings are you actually consuming? Very important to look at serving size - often you eat or drink the entire contents of the container and it may be 2 or 3 times what you think you are consuming. If in fact the label reads "Serving Per Container 2," it is best to portion out the food or drink and save the other half for later.

Calories: Eating too many calories per day is linked to weight gain and observing this part of the label is very helpful in gaining, losing and maintaining. Look carefully at the label below - you may be tricked into thinking there are 250 calories in this product, but in fact because the servings per container is "2" - the total calories would be a shocking 500 with 220 coming from fat.

Nutrition Facts
Serving Size 1 cup (228g)
Servings Per Container 2

Amount Per Serving

Calories 250	Calories from Fat 110

	% Daily Value
Total Fat 12g	18%
Saturated Fat 3g	15%
Trans Fat 3g	
Cholesterol 30mg	10%
Sodium 47mg	20%
Potassium 700mg	20%
Total Carbohydrate 31g	10%
Dietary Fiber 0g	0%
Sugars 5g	
Protein 5g	
Vitamin A	4%
Vitamin C	2%
Calcium	20%
Iron	4%

*Precent Daily Values are based on a 2,000 calori diet. Your Daily Value may be higher or lower depending on your calorie needs.

	Calories	2,000	2500
Total Fat:	Less Than	65g	80g
Sat Fat:	Less Than	20g	25g
Cholesterol	Less Than	300mg	300mg
Sodium	Less Than	2400mg	2,400mg
Total Carbohydrates		300g	375g
Dietary Fiber		25g	30g

A General Guide to Caloric Intake:
- 40 Calories is Low
- 100 Calories is Moderate
- 400 Calories is High

Fiber: An important element to have in your diet and one of the few nutrients found on the food label that you want to be high. It's helpful in the reduction of many health risks. Good sources of fiber include high fiber cereal such as shredded wheat and whole grain raisin bran. Fruits such as berries, raisins and bananas, as well as whole grain breads and pastas.

Look for fiber when buying bread, cereal, or pasta; you want to see at least 2 grams of fiber per serving. The more fiber your food contains, the fuller you will feel after eating it. You need at least 25 grams daily.

Carbohydrates: There are 2 types of carbs- simple (white bread, white rice, chips, cookies, candy and junk food) and complex (oatmeal, beans, whole wheat flour, sweet potatoes and most other fruits and veggies.) If a food has a good amount of fiber, it's most likely a complex carb; if it has a good amount of sugar, it's most likely a simple carb.

Protein: Contains 4 calories per gram. Protein plays an important role in muscle, cell, organ and gland function. Some examples of high protein foods include meat, fish, chicken, turkey, nuts and seeds.

Sugar: It is often listed in "alias" terms like high fructose corn syrup, dextrose, or turbinado. Try to choose foods with less than 5 grams of sugar per serving.

Salt: Another name for salt is sodium and it should be restricted to 2300 mg per day (which is less than one tsp. of salt). To reduce your salt intake, choose less processed foods & beverages.

Hint: Read the front of a food package. Very often creative advertisers will use phrases like "reduced fat" or "smart choice" - it is not necessarily a healthier choice. In 1990 the Nutrition Labeling and Education Act (NLEA) required all packaged foods to list nutritional ingredients. Manufacturers are required to list all ingredients contained in the product by weight. It is best to be able to read and pronounce all of the ingredients; products with fewer ingredients are usually healthier.

Let's Find Out Where You Are!

1. Do you eat at least one piece of raw fruit every day? **Yes   No**
2. Do you eat breakfast? ("just coffee" doesn't count!) **Yes   No**
3. Do you eat at least 3 servings of vegetables daily? **Yes   No**
4. Do you include fish in your diet at least two times a week? **Yes   No**
5. Do you chew your food thoroughly? **Yes   No**
6. Do you drink at least 8 glasses of filtered or spring water every day? **Yes   No**
7. Do you avoid beer, alcohol, and soda while eating? **Yes   No**
8. If you are stressed or upset, do you wait for the feeling to pass before you eat? **Yes   No**
9. Do you drink raw vegetable juice at least once a week? **Yes   No**
10. Do you avoid foods that contain sugar? **Yes   No**

Your Score: Add up your Yes answers

★★★ **7 - 10 Excellent**
You have a good handle on the nutrition necessary for a healthy diet

★★ **4 - 6 Good, but Room for Improvement**
You are probably trying hard to eat the right foods; it will get easier when it becomes a habit.

★ **1 - 3 Uh Oh!**
You have some work to do, but we are here to help!

Personal Stats
At the start of your journey

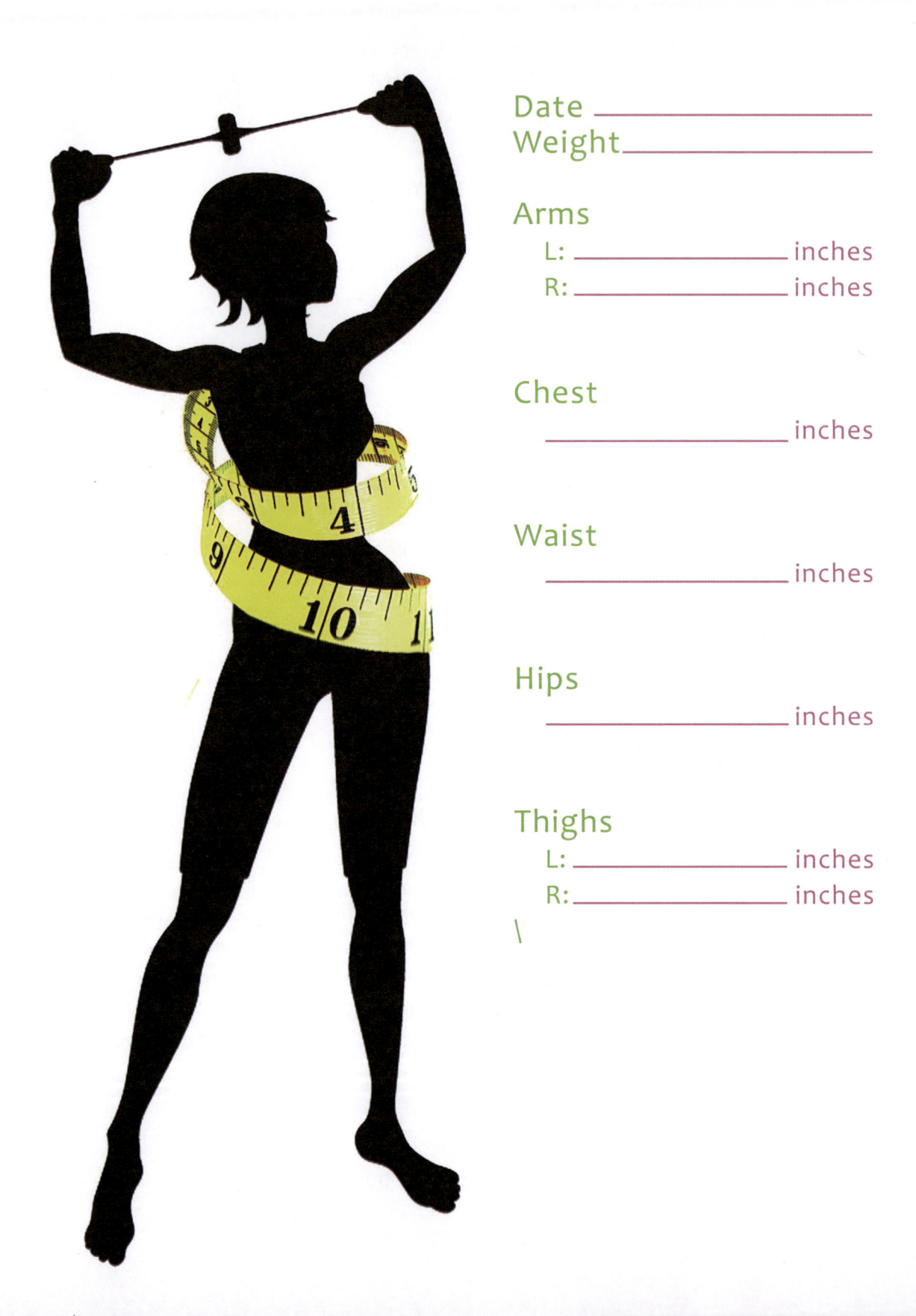

Date _____
Weight_____

Arms
    L: _____ inches
    R: _____ inches

Chest
_____ inches

Waist
_____ inches

Hips
_____ inches

Thighs
    L: _____ inches
    R: _____ inches

Before Photo

Wear shorts and a tight shirt. Don't be afraid to let it all hang out. Things will get better!

Inspiration Photo

Find an ideal body type (in a magazine) that inspires you towards your goal!

What I Eat

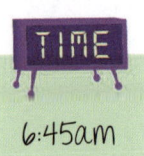

Week 1 — **Day 1**

6:45am — Upon Rising: 2 oz Paul Bragg's Apple Cider Vinegar mixed with 6 oz warm water

7:30am — Breakfast: 3 scrambled egg whites mixed with 1/2 cup raw spinach, 3/4 cup diced onion, 1 slice multi-grain bread, 1 cup hot green tea

10:20am — Snack: 6 large strawberries, 6 oz plain non-fat Greek yogurt, a handful of raw almonds and half an apple

12:15pm — Lunch: 4 oz grilled chicken breast
salad: 2 cups romaine lettuce, 3/4 cup mushrooms, 1/2 sliced tomato, 1/4 cup shredded carrots, 3 kalamatta olives + 2 tsp balsamic vinaigrette

4:00pm — Snack: berry smoothie
2 cups frozen blueberries/strawberries, 1 scoop low calorie whey protein powder, 1 tbsp flaxseed oil, 1 tsp chia seeds

7:00pm — Dinner: 6 oz grilled wild salmon, 1 cup sauteed green beans, 1/2 baked sweet potato,
salad: 1 cup spring mixed lettuce, 1/4 tomato, 1/4 cup green pepper, 1/4 cup yellow pepper, 1/2 oz almonds, 1 tsp. balsamic vinaigrette

8:10pm — Snack: 1 cup low-fat cottage cheese mixed with 2 slivers of fresh peaches and a light sprinkle of cinnamon

Place a check on the water cups to keep track of every 8oz you drink

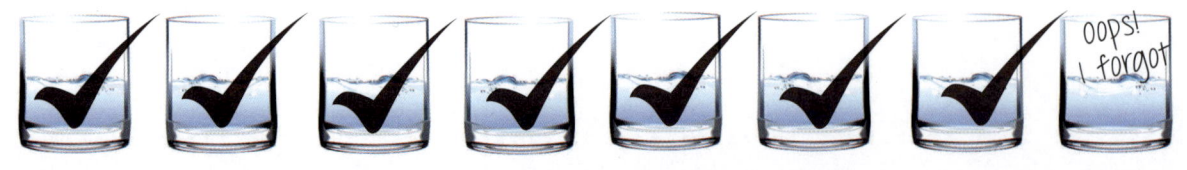

✓ ✓ ✓ ✓ ✓ ✓ ✓ oops! I forgot

This is what I ate on March 20th...

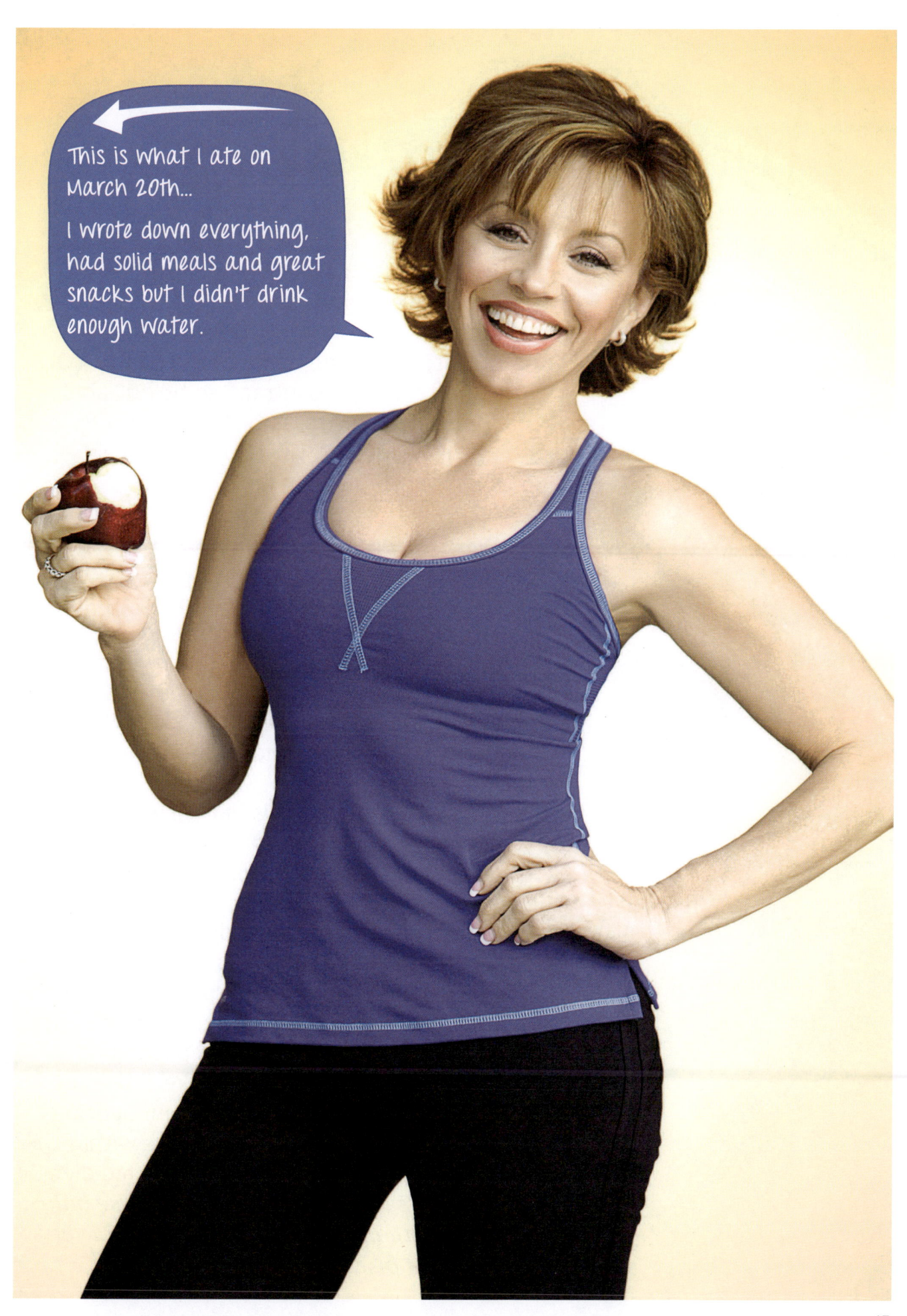

I wrote down everything, had solid meals and great snacks but I didn't drink enough water.

Now Remember

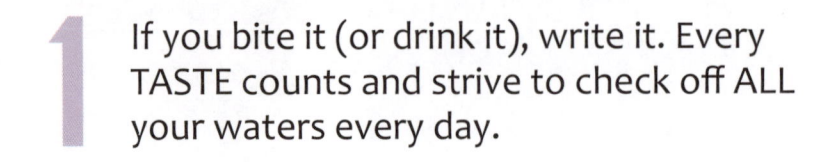

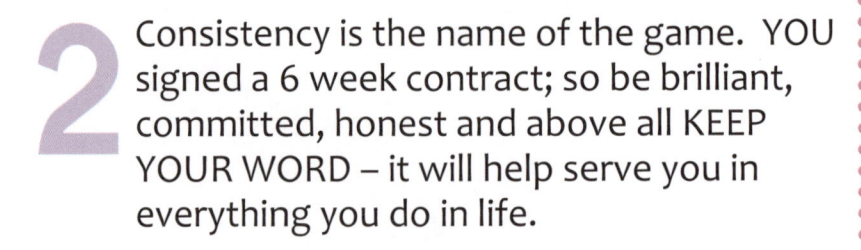

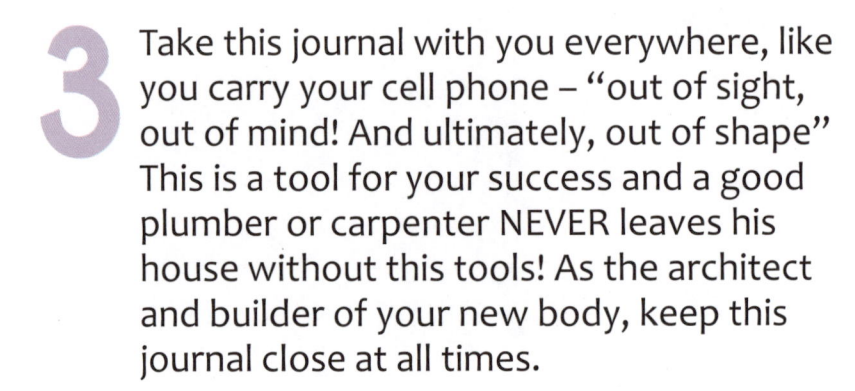

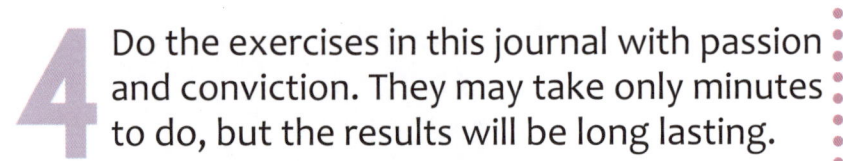

1 If you bite it (or drink it), write it. Every TASTE counts and strive to check off ALL your waters every day.

2 Consistency is the name of the game. YOU signed a 6 week contract; so be brilliant, committed, honest and above all KEEP YOUR WORD – it will help serve you in everything you do in life.

3 Take this journal with you everywhere, like you carry your cell phone – "out of sight, out of mind! And ultimately, out of shape" This is a tool for your success and a good plumber or carpenter NEVER leaves his house without this tools! As the architect and builder of your new body, keep this journal close at all times.

4 Do the exercises in this journal with passion and conviction. They may take only minutes to do, but the results will be long lasting.

5 Lastly, you are NOT on a diet. Don't restrict your food intake or make radical changes. The beginning part of this program is simply for you to see what you eat, when you eat and why you eat. The act of becoming aware of your daily food intake and your behavior has a magical way of influencing both. You'll make subtle changes within yourself, without ever going on a fad diet again. *A sailboat that changes course but one degree, over time will end up in a very different place... and so will you.*

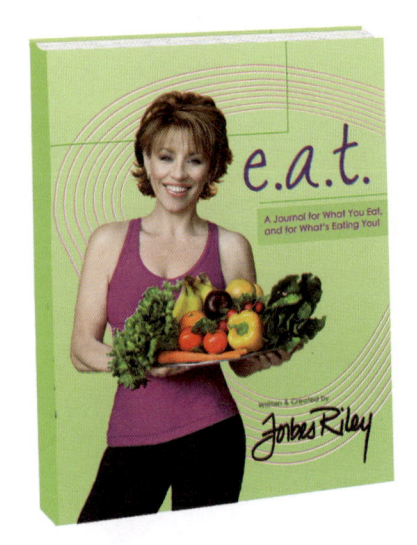

I believe in you, so let's get ready to e.a.t.

Week 1

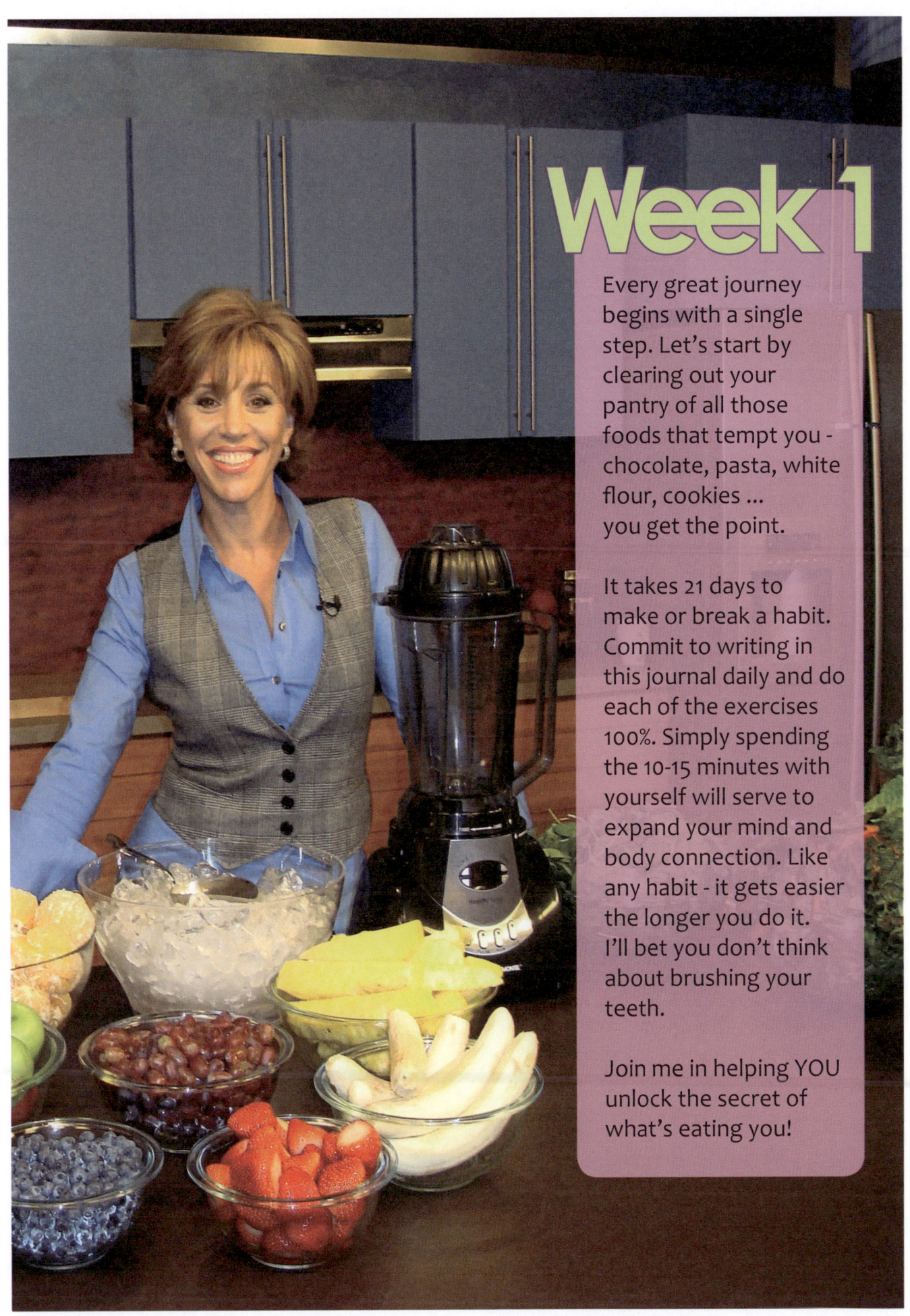

Every great journey begins with a single step. Let's start by clearing out your pantry of all those foods that tempt you - chocolate, pasta, white flour, cookies ... you get the point.

It takes 21 days to make or break a habit. Commit to writing in this journal daily and do each of the exercises 100%. Simply spending the 10-15 minutes with yourself will serve to expand your mind and body connection. Like any habit - it gets easier the longer you do it. I'll bet you don't think about brushing your teeth.

Join me in helping YOU unlock the secret of what's eating you!

What I Eat

Week 1 **Day 1**

TIME

Upon Rising

Breakfast

Snack

Lunch

Snack

Dinner

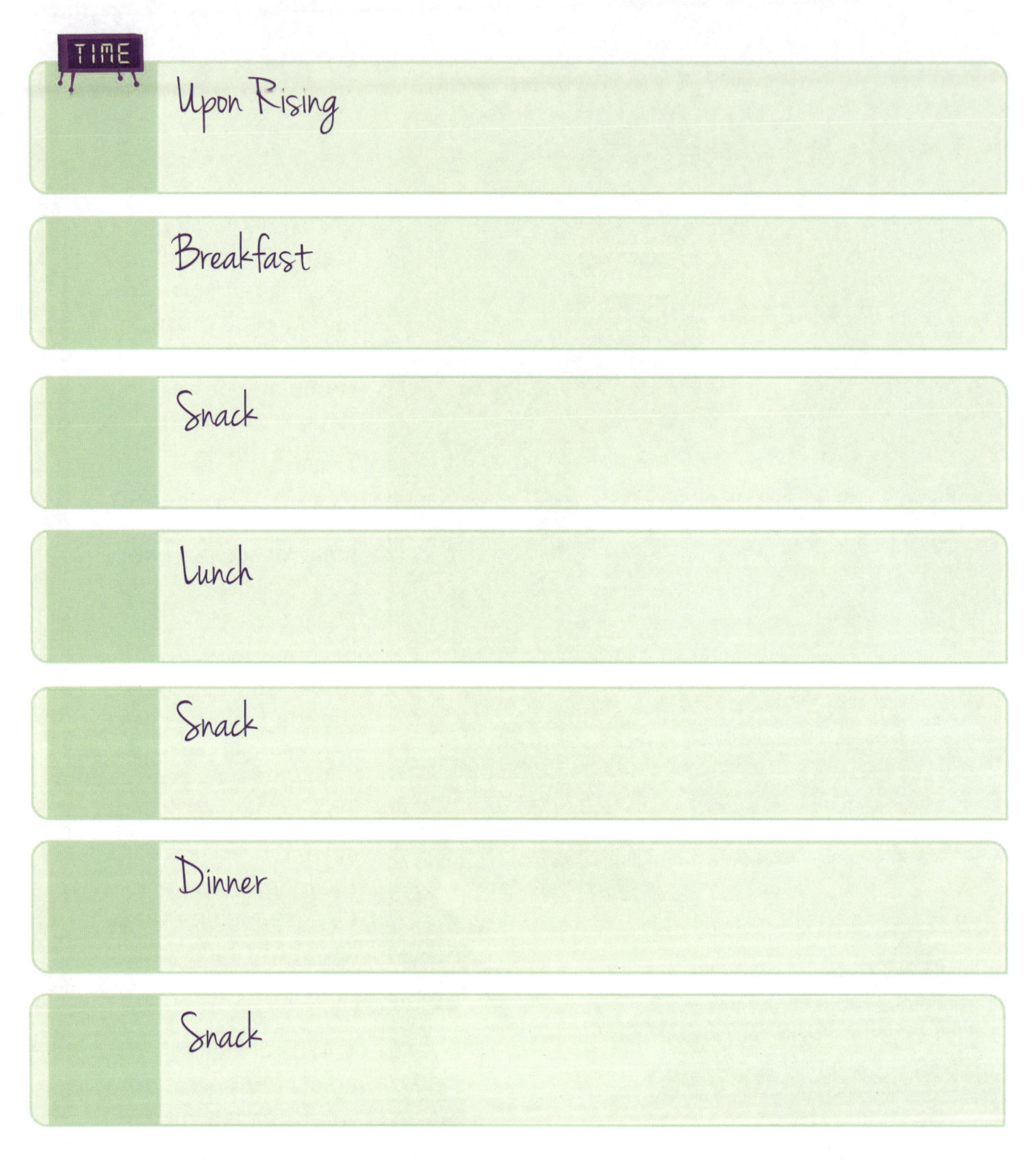

Snack

Place a check on the water cups to keep track of every 8oz you drink

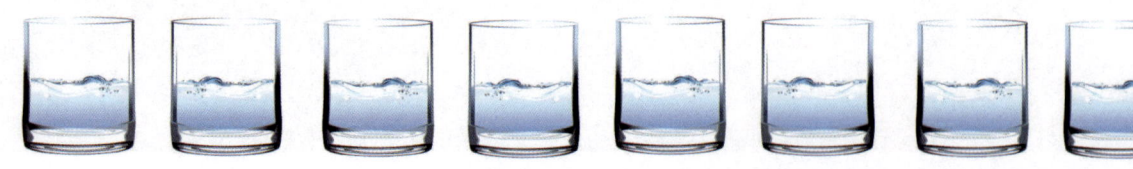

Ready, Set, Go!
Write down everything you're thinking and feeling right now.

**No Editing...
Unload your fears, hopes and goals!**

"Leap and the net will appear!"

What I Eat

Week 1 · Day 2

TIME

Upon Rising

Breakfast

Snack

Lunch

Snack

Dinner

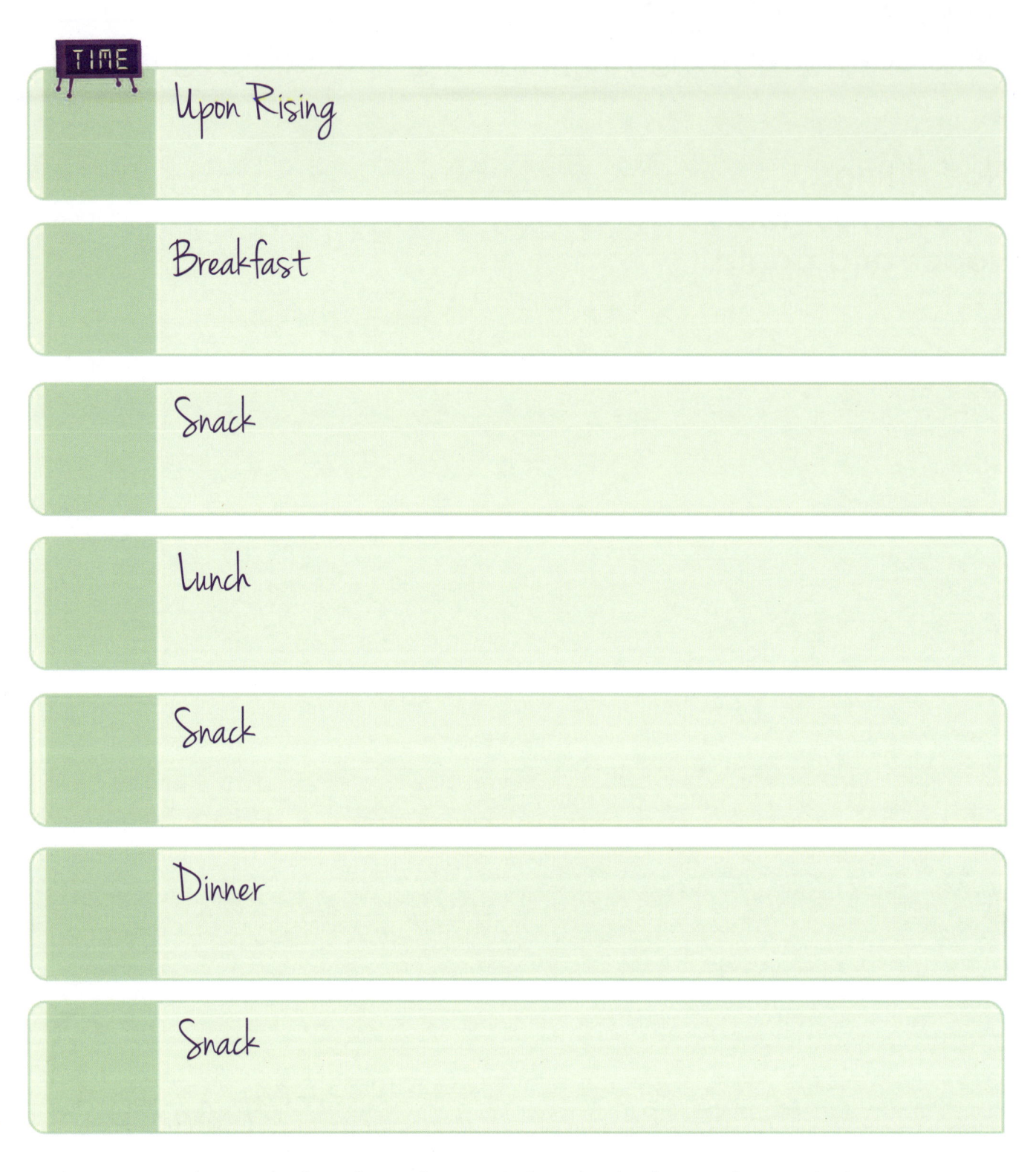

Snack

Place a check on the water cups to keep track of every 8oz you drink

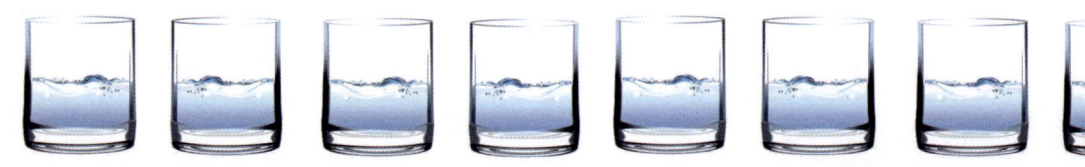

Commit (kuh-mit) verb

1. To pledge or engage one's self (an athlete commits to the highest standards)
2. To bind or obligate (to commit one's self to a promise or course of action)

What are 3 things you're committed to achieving this week and why?

1

2

3

> **TIP**
> Vitamins are complex substances that are essential for good body functions. In order to get all the vitamins we need from foods, we would have to eat at least 5 cups of fruit and veggies per day... Did you??? Take your vitamins daily.

Week 1 — What I Eat — **Day 3**

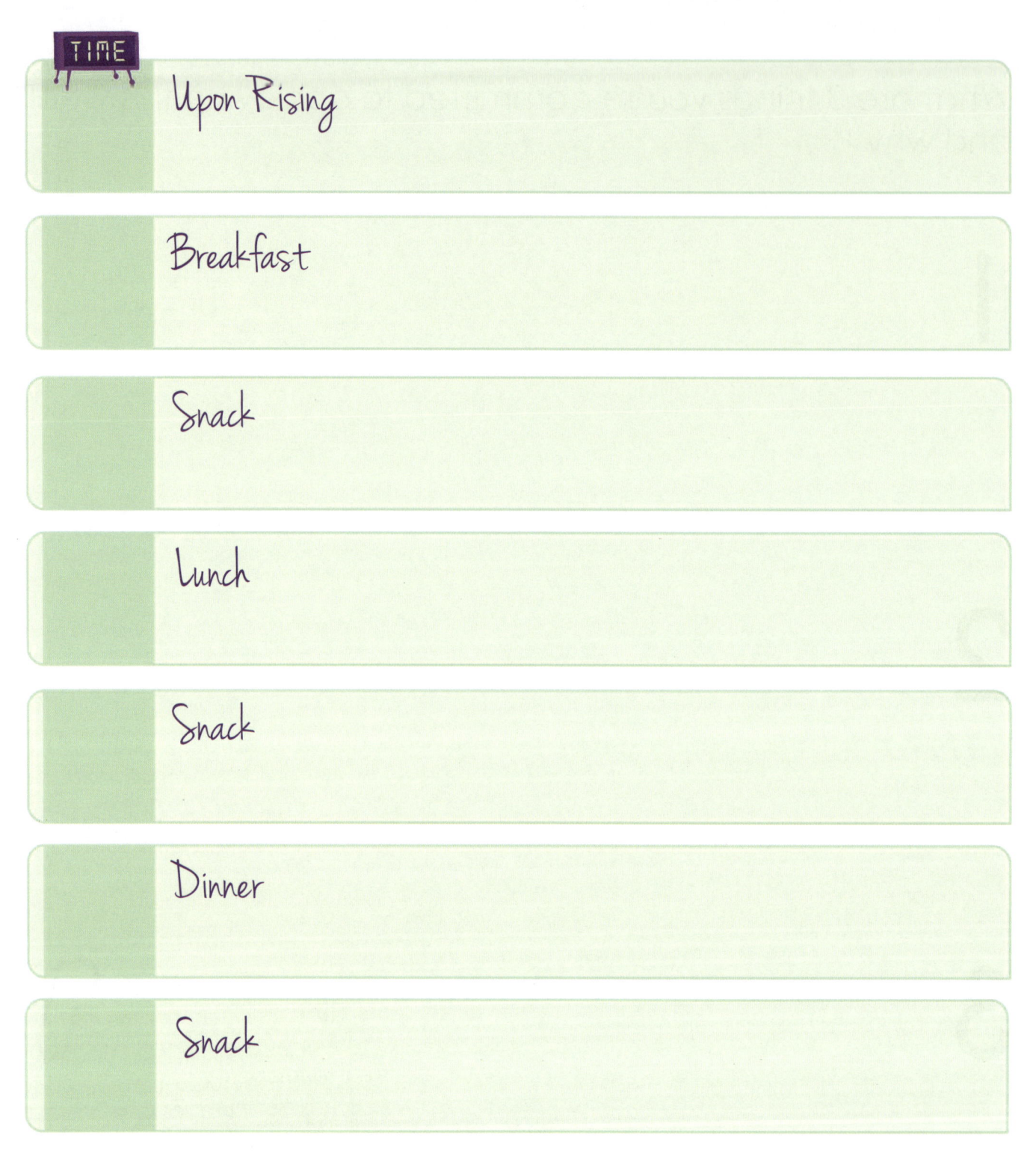

TIME

- Upon Rising
- Breakfast
- Snack
- Lunch
- Snack
- Dinner
- Snack

Place a check on the water cups to keep track of every 8oz you drink

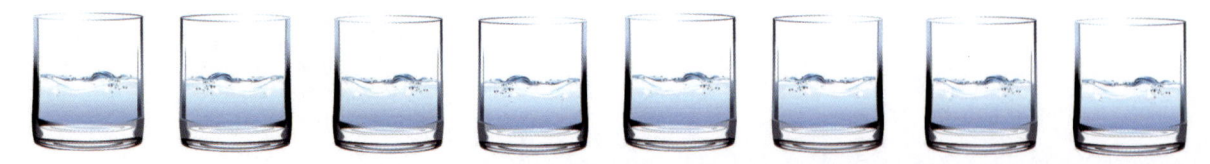

Write down **5 things** that make you happy, and why.

1 _____

2 _____

3 _____

4 _____

5 _____

For a mood Shifter

Try smiling even when you don't feel like it!

TIP
Add music.

Music makes you want to move. It makes time fly, so listen to your favorite tunes and dance in your house or wear headphones when you walk or workout. Burn those extra calories.

Week 1 # What I Eat **Day 4**

TIME

Upon Rising

Breakfast

Snack

Lunch

Snack

Dinner

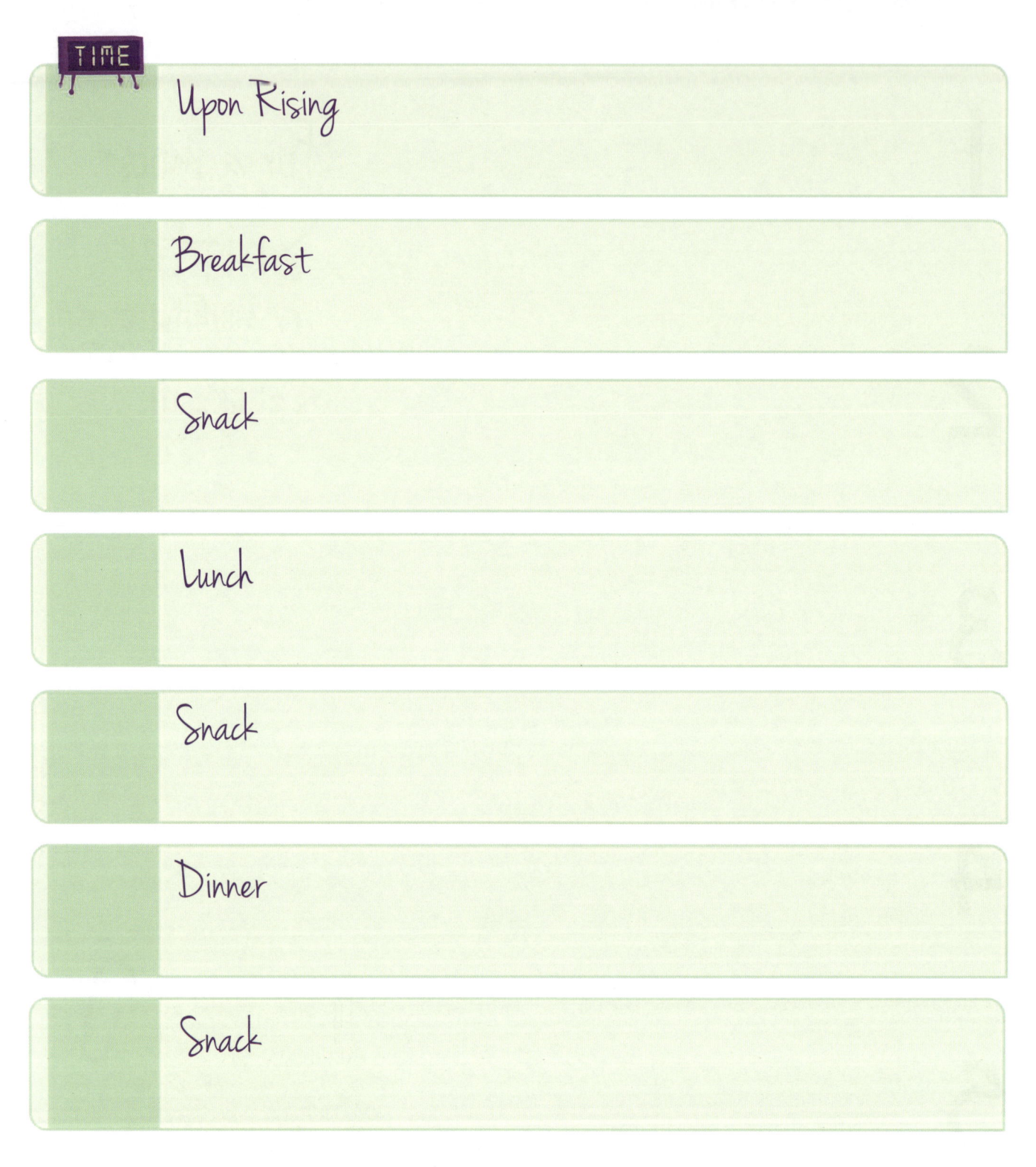

Snack

Place a check on the water cups to keep track of every 8oz you drink

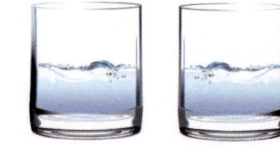

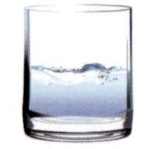

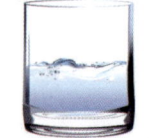

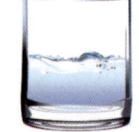

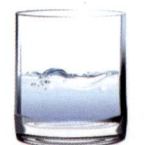

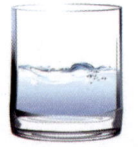

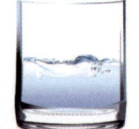

Time Travel

Remember yourself as a young child. What did you like to do? What were your favorite things to play with? As your inner child, write a letter to yourself at your age today. What were your hopes and dreams? What would you tell yourself now?

Dear

Love Me

What I Eat

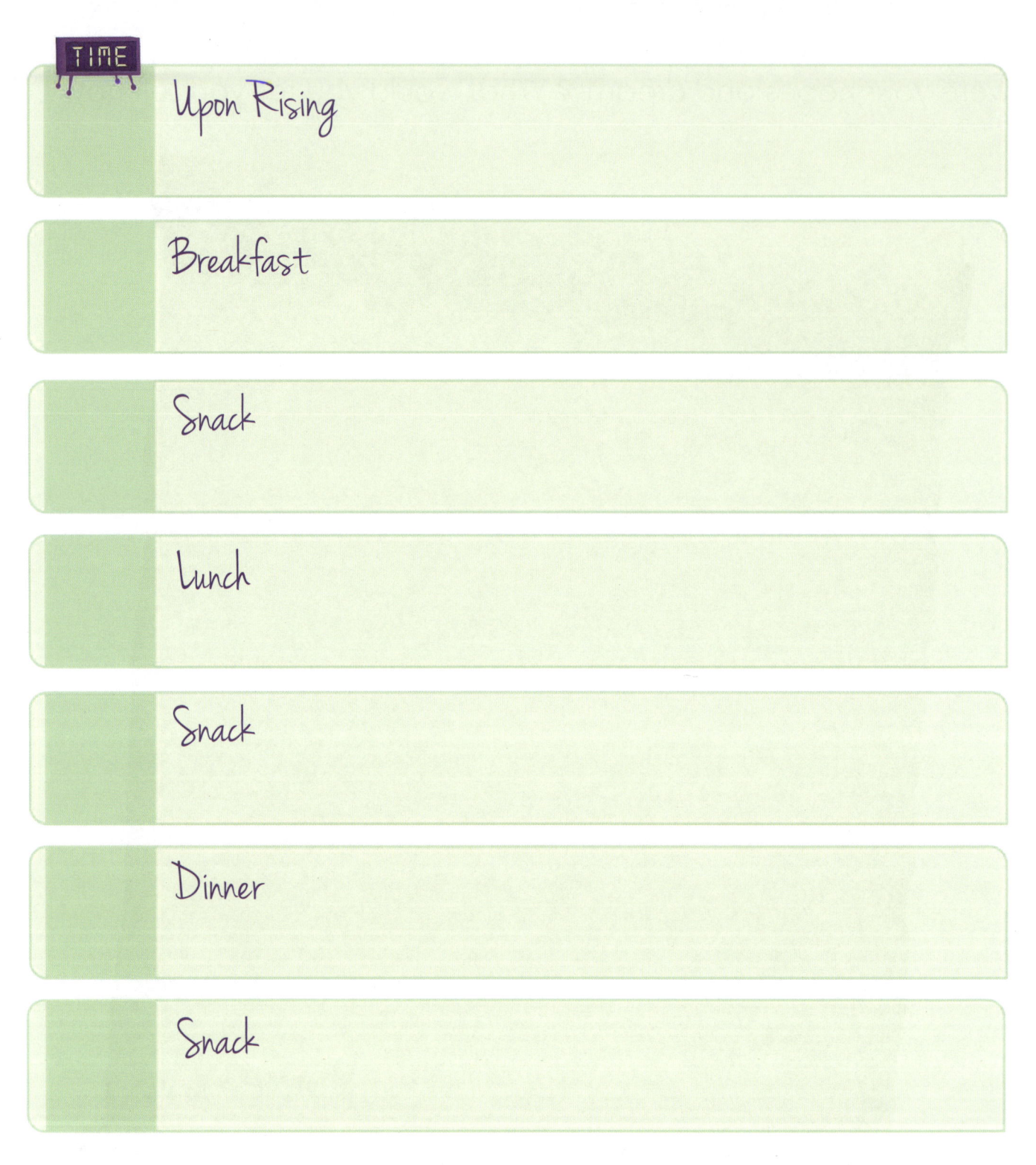

Week 1 — **Day 5**

TIME

- Upon Rising
- Breakfast
- Snack
- Lunch
- Snack
- Dinner
- Snack

Place a check on the water cups to keep track of every 8oz you drink

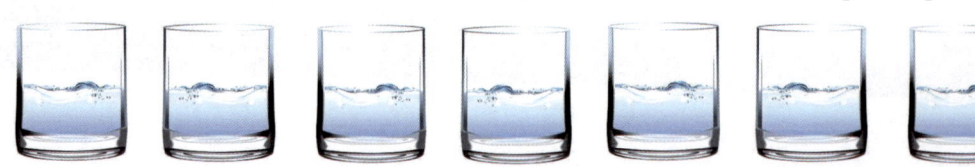

Beautiful (byoo-tuh-fuh-l) Adjective

1. Possessing beauty; having qualities that give great pleasure or satisfaction to see, hear, think about, etc.; delighting the senses or mind. *The flowers were especially beautiful this year.*
2. Stands out from the rest. *It was beautiful to watch her dance.*

Write down 5 things in your life that are beautiful and excite your senses to see, feel, touch, or smell.

1.

2.

3.

4.

5.

TIP

At restaurants, pass on the bread basket. It may be tempting to eat, but while on this 6 week program ask the waiter to take it away and start with a soup or salad instead. Also, think twice; do you really need that dessert?

Remember, desserts is stressed spelled backwards.

What I Eat

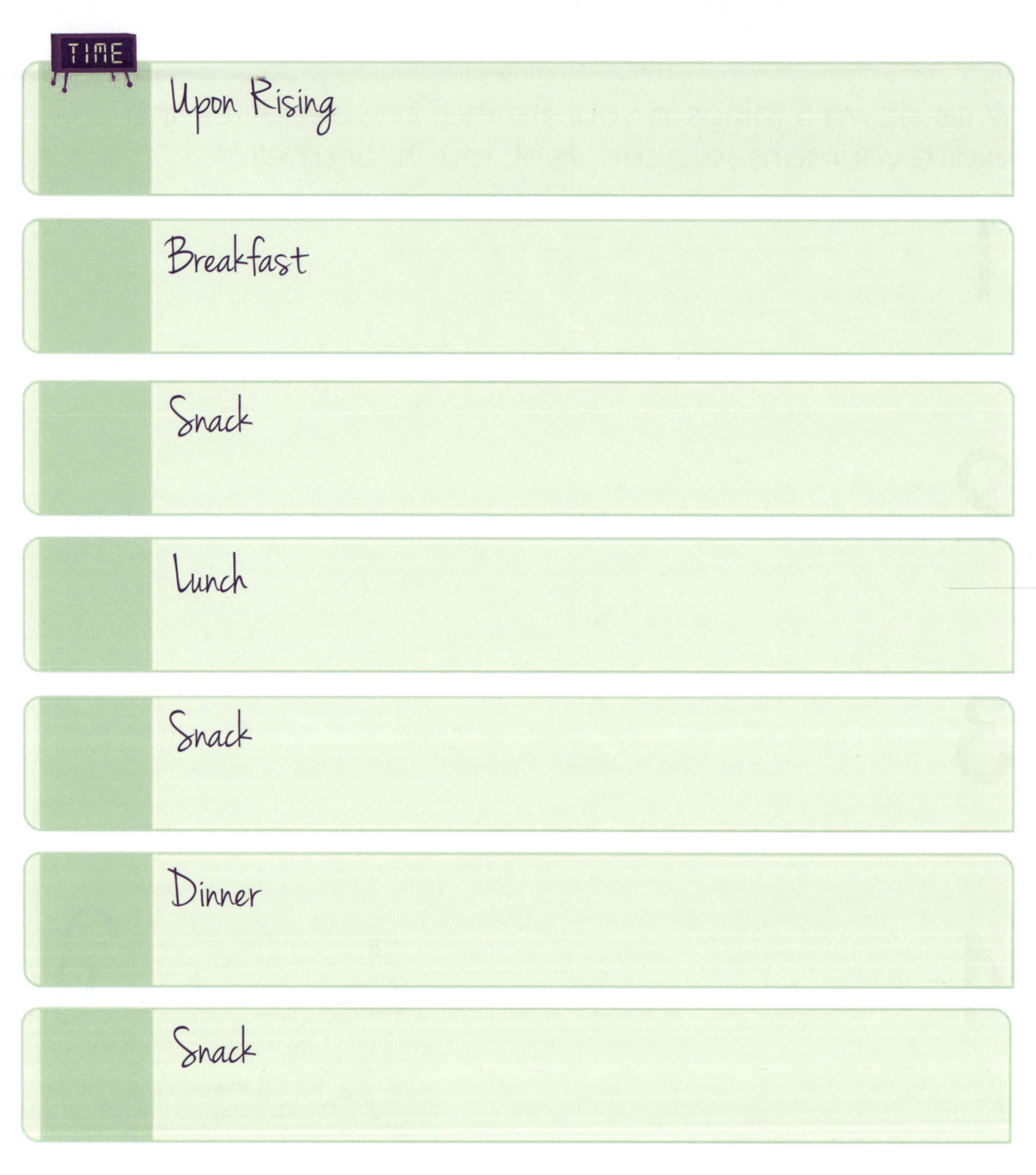

Week 1 — **Day 6**

TIME

- Upon Rising
- Breakfast
- Snack
- Lunch
- Snack
- Dinner
- Snack

Place a check on the water cups to keep track of every 8oz you drink

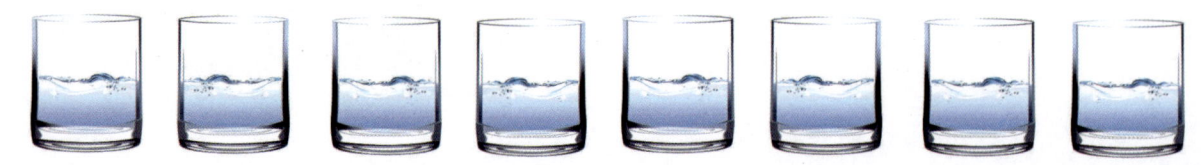

Imagine your perfect vacation, anywhere around the world

If you could have a *magic wand* and travel anywhere in the world you've ever dreamed of - where would it be? Imagine the perfect vacation there and describe in detail.

TIP

Clean out the clutter. Start small. Organize your purse, wallet, briefcase or tote bag. Clutter drains your energy. Even the tiniest changes help to produce more vitality in your world.

What I Eat

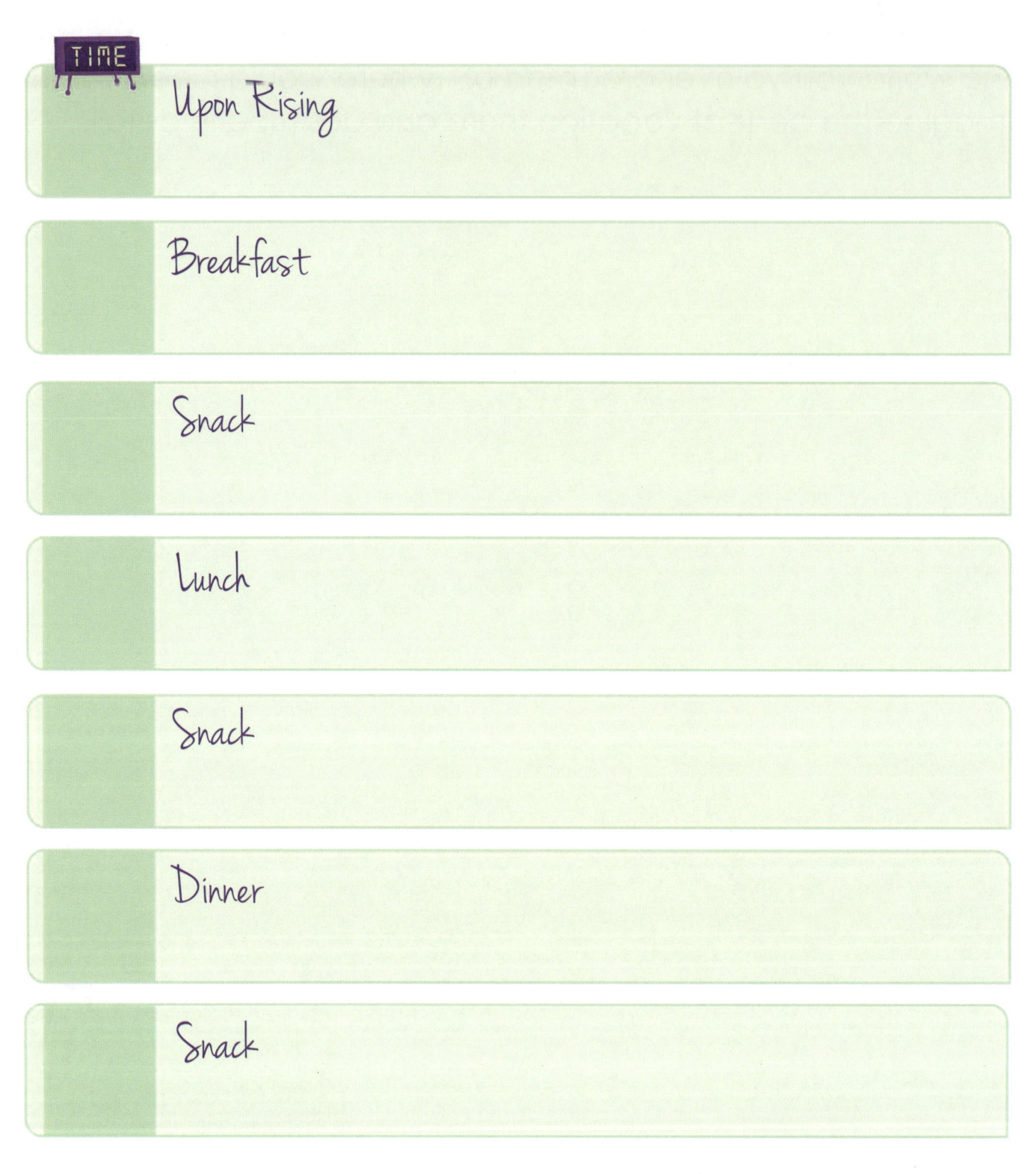

Week 1   **Day 7**

TIME

- Upon Rising
- Breakfast
- Snack
- Lunch
- Snack
- Dinner
- Snack

Place a check on the water cups to keep track of every 8oz you drink

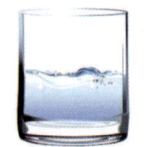

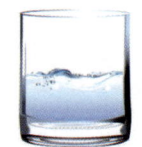

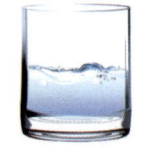

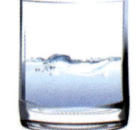

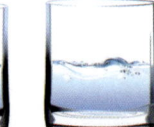

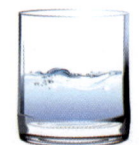

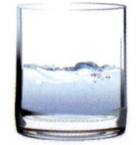

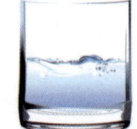

Congrats! You have made it to the end of the 1st week. Time to check in with yourself.

1 How many days this week did you fill in your journal? Write the number, not the excuses.

Fill in the number of days be honest!

2 Biggest obstacles this week:
List strategies for overcoming them.

....
....
....
....
....
....

3 What are your goals for the future?

....
....
....
....
....
....

Top 10 Superfoods

Now that you have observed the foods you typically eat in a week, let's try introducing some high nutrient, low calorie SUPERFOODS.

This week, try to incorporate at least 3 to 4 of the following into your daily meal plan.

Broccoli
Shaped like a tree and best served when it's bright green. Broccoli goes nice with meat, chicken and fish. One serving contains more vitamin C than a glass of orange juice. Best prep methods: raw, steaming, microwave or stir fry. Boiling is not recommended, as it destroys the nutrients.

Wild Salmon
Is a nutrient dense source of proteins, vitamins and minerals. The fats found in this fish are high in EFA (Essential Fatty Acids), which are essential for keeping body tissue healthy. Wild salmon is preferred over farm raised.

Quinoa (pronounced *keen-wah*)
One of the best whole grains you can eat. High in protein; 8 grams in one cooked cup. 5 grams per cup of fiber and a great source of iron. Quinoa is also loaded with plenty of zinc, vitamin E and selenium. Quinoa is as easy to prepare as rice. It can be eaten alone or mixed with vegetables, nuts, or lean protein.

Spinach
Popeye loved it for a good reason. It is perfect for salads, wraps, soups and omelettes. Contains an abundance of vitamins A, B6, C, E, and K. Also includes minerals iron, calcium, magnesium and zinc. Excellent vegetable eaten raw, steamed, or sauteed. Did you know that one cup of cooked spinach has 5 grams of protein.

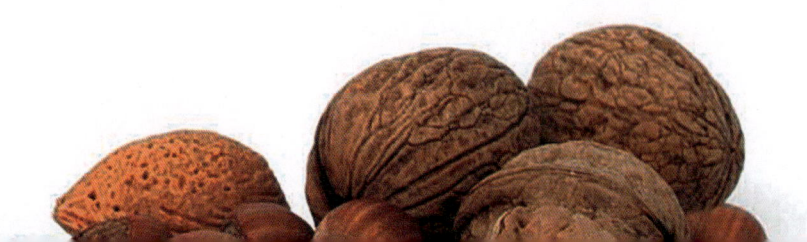

Oatmeal
One of the few foods rich in silicon, a mineral responsible for building beautiful skin, hair, bones and teeth. Steel cut oatmeal is a slow burning complex carbohydrate that promotes the feeling of fullness and prevents the spiking of blood sugars. A bowl of hot oatmeal is one of the best ways to start your day.

Soy
The soybean is actually a legume, but is in a class all of its own because it contains many nutrients. Believed by many to be a source of complete proteins. An excellent source of zinc, potassium, B vitamins, as well as a soluble fiber and omega 3 fatty acids.

Eggs
They make the list because they are nutritious, versatile, economical and a great source of quality protein. They contain 12 vitamins and minerals, including choline, for brain development and memory. Boiled, scrambled, or even lightly fried - try eating eggs for a meal other than breakfast, you'll be surprised.

Nuts
Many people shy away from nuts because of their high fat content. However, they are chock full of protein, high in fiber and anti-oxidants. The key to enjoying nuts is portion control - all nuts are healthy in small doses. Almonds are a rich source of vitamin E, peanuts contain resveratrol also found in red grapes and wine and Brazil nuts are one of the richest sources of the antioxidant selenium. Sprinkle on your cereal, add to your yogurt or just snack right out of the bag.

Blueberries
Are power packed with enormous quantities of anti-oxidants and fiber. They are loaded with iron, vitamins A, C, B6 and anthocyanin. Best eaten hot or cold in smoothies, muffins or in a salad. Blueberries are a must for a healthy diet.

Beans
Beans are loaded with fiber, vegetable protein and vitamins. Best to soak them overnight. Try hummus or bean spreads instead of fatty dips made with sour cream or mayonnaise.
To spice up your favorite dishes, incorporate beans into soups, salads and stews. Choose from black, pinto, navy, kidney, lima, soy and garbanzo.

Fun & Healthy e.a.t. Recipe #1

Blueberry Muffins

Blueberries are a healthy choice and a good source of antioxidants, great eaten raw, but as a muffin - watch out! The blueberry muffins found in today's bakery cases are not healthy. Did you know that muffins sold today in coffee shops and grocery stores are more than twice as big as those sold in the 1950's and more than 3 times the size of one standard portion?

At a popular coffee house, blueberry muffins pack a whopping 450 calories, 22 grams of fat and 31 grams of sugar. This is where healthy blueberry muffins come in!

The e.a.t. Healthy Alternative
196 calories, 5.8 grams of fat, and 15 grams of sugar

Ingredients

1 cup fresh blueberries
3/4 cup whole-wheat flour
3/4 cup all-purpose flour
1/4 cup oat bran
1/4 cup quick cooking oats
One egg
1 cup low fat Greek yogurt (plain)
3/4 cup organic apple sauce
1 tsp baking powder
1 tsp baking soda
1 tsp vanilla
One good pinch of salt
3/4 cup fructose

1 Preheat oven to 350 degrees. Spray muffin pan with non-stick cooking spray or line with paper muffin cups.

2 Blend applesauce, yogurt, vanilla, and egg in bowl and set aside. Stir flour, fructose, baking powder, baking soda, oats and salt in a medium bowl.

3 Pour wet ingredients into the center of the dry ingredient bowl and stir until the flour is moistened. Fold in blueberries, stir again, but do not over mix.

4 Divide batter among muffin cups and bake until golden brown, approximately 18 - 20 minutes. *Makes 12 muffins.*

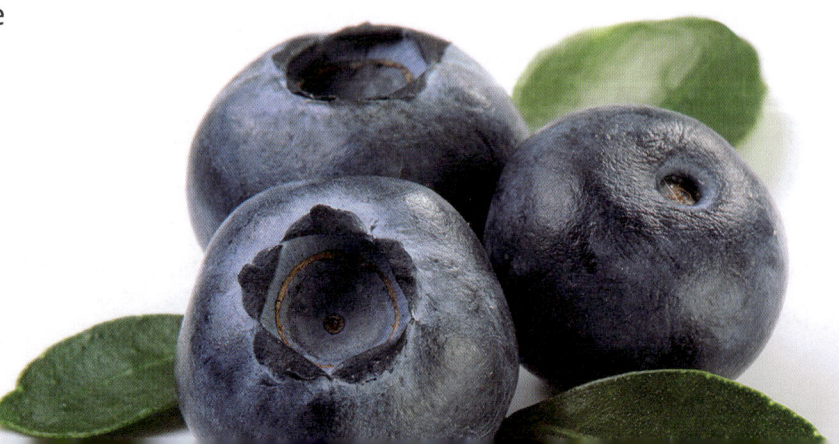

Forbes Fit & Fun

I've included some games throughout this journal for those moments when you're stuck waiting at a restaurant, airport, or any place you might be tempted to eat the wrong food. Take a moment and make great choices. Are you ready for week 2?

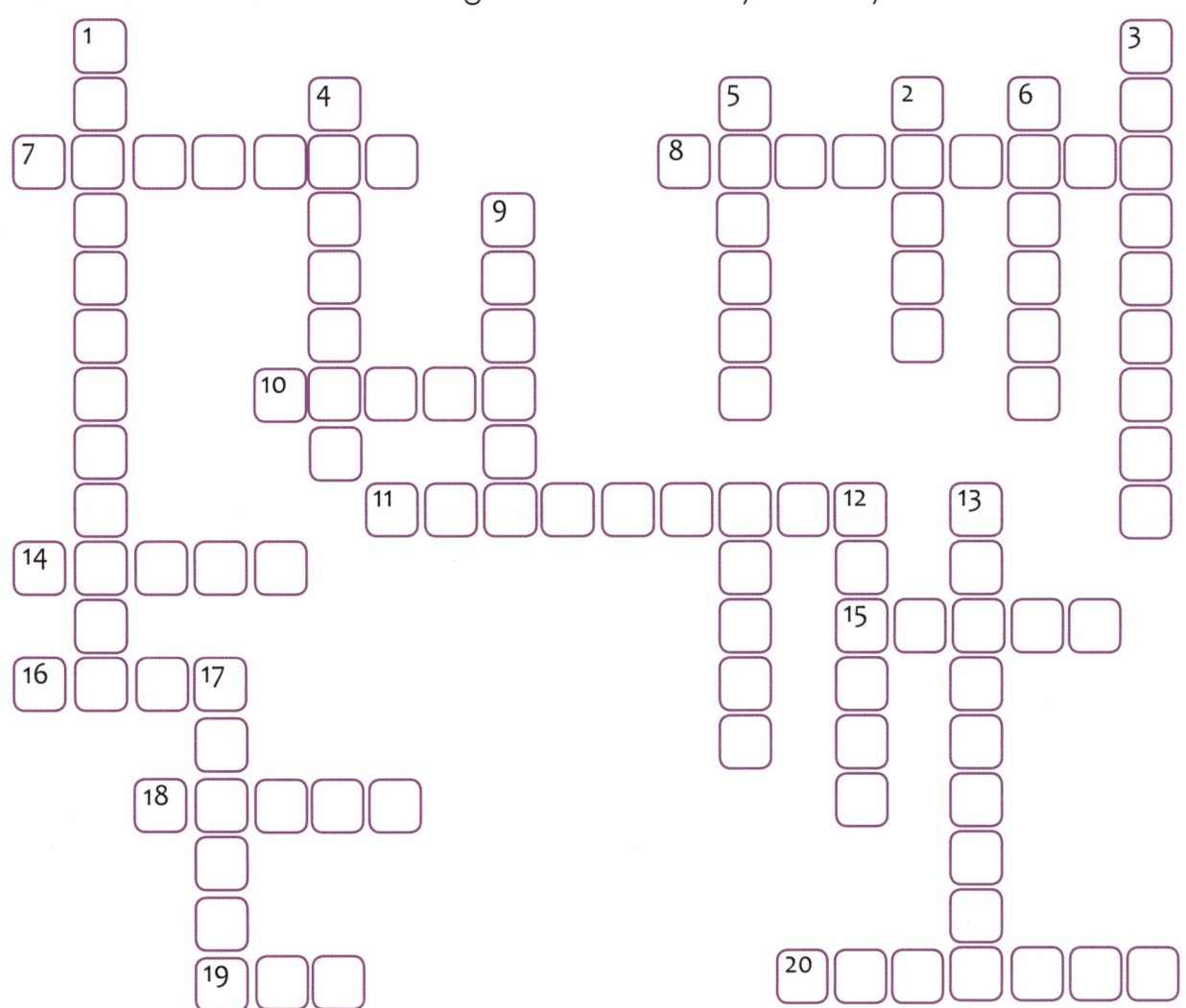

Across

7. An egg is a form of _____
8. A dieters worst night of the year!
10. The largest bone in the body
11. A type of "not so smart" free weight
14. Everywhere but not a drop to drink
15. To rid your body of toxins and chemicals
16. A calorie is a measure of this
18. Wheat, rye, barley
19. The most important person
20. Forbes Riley favorite piece of fitness equipment

Down

1. A slice of bread is a form of _____
2. She looks amazing in leg warmers
3. Good nutrition helps to improve your body's _____
4. A unique form of exercise that focuses on the "Powerhouse," often done on a reformer
5. The Grandfather of fitness
6. A state of physical, social & mental well-being
9. Yoga done in a very HOT room!
12. Another name for salt
13. The science of food.

Notes

> Many of life's failures are people who didn't realize how close they were to success when they gave up.
>
> — Thomas Edison

Week 2

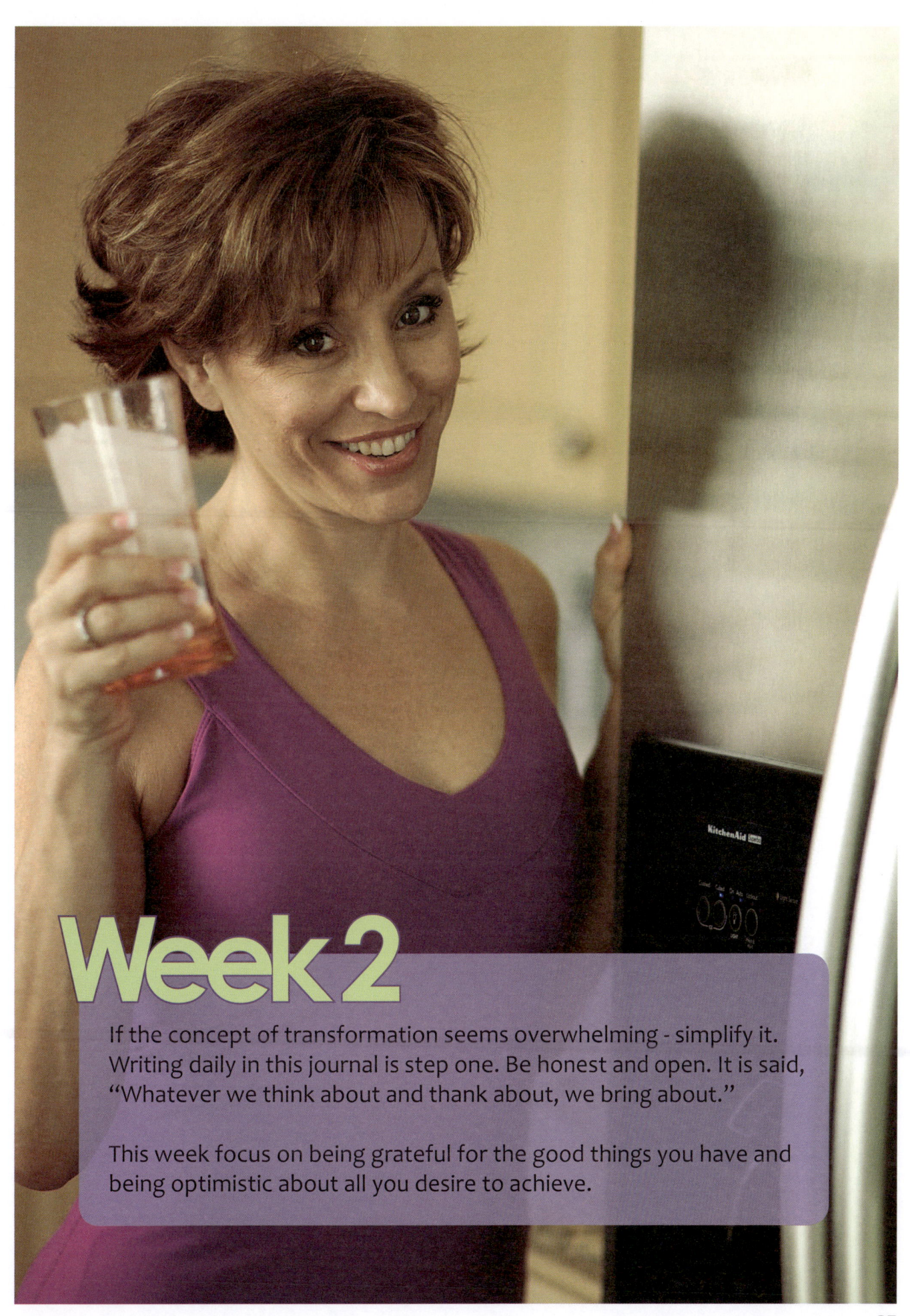

If the concept of transformation seems overwhelming - simplify it. Writing daily in this journal is step one. Be honest and open. It is said, "Whatever we think about and thank about, we bring about."

This week focus on being grateful for the good things you have and being optimistic about all you desire to achieve.

Week 2 # What I Eat **Day 1**

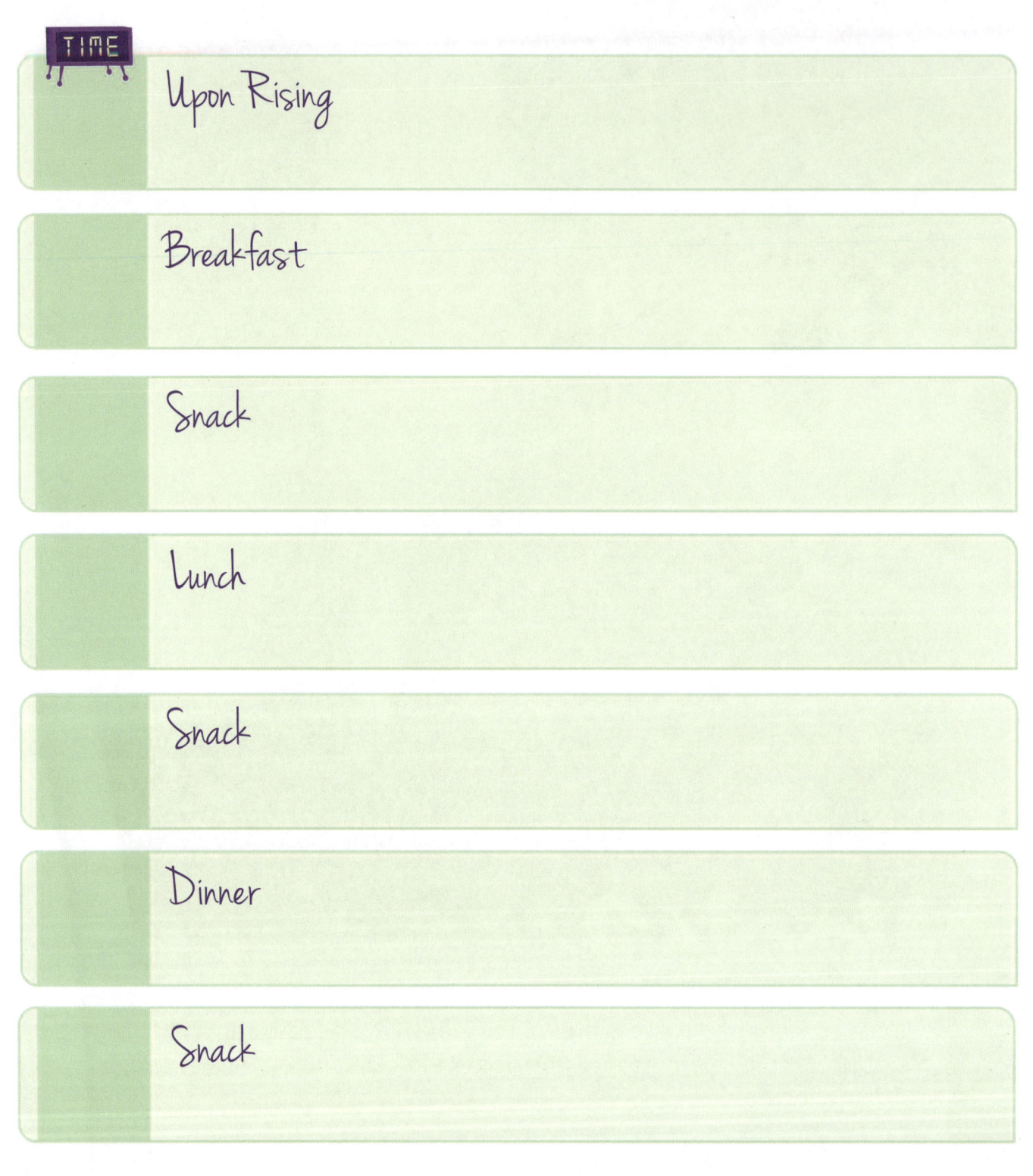

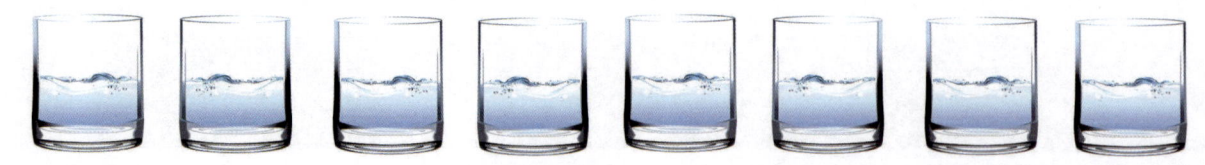

TIME

Upon Rising

Breakfast

Snack

Lunch

Snack

Dinner

Snack

Place a check on the water cups to keep track of every 8oz you drink

Ready, Set, Write!

Let's start this week with exercise, (I recommend you incorporate some physical activity daily: walking, swimming, SpinGym, etc.) but on this page the, "exercise" is to stretch your creativity and imagination. Spend the next few minutes freely writing all of the thoughts that come into your head.

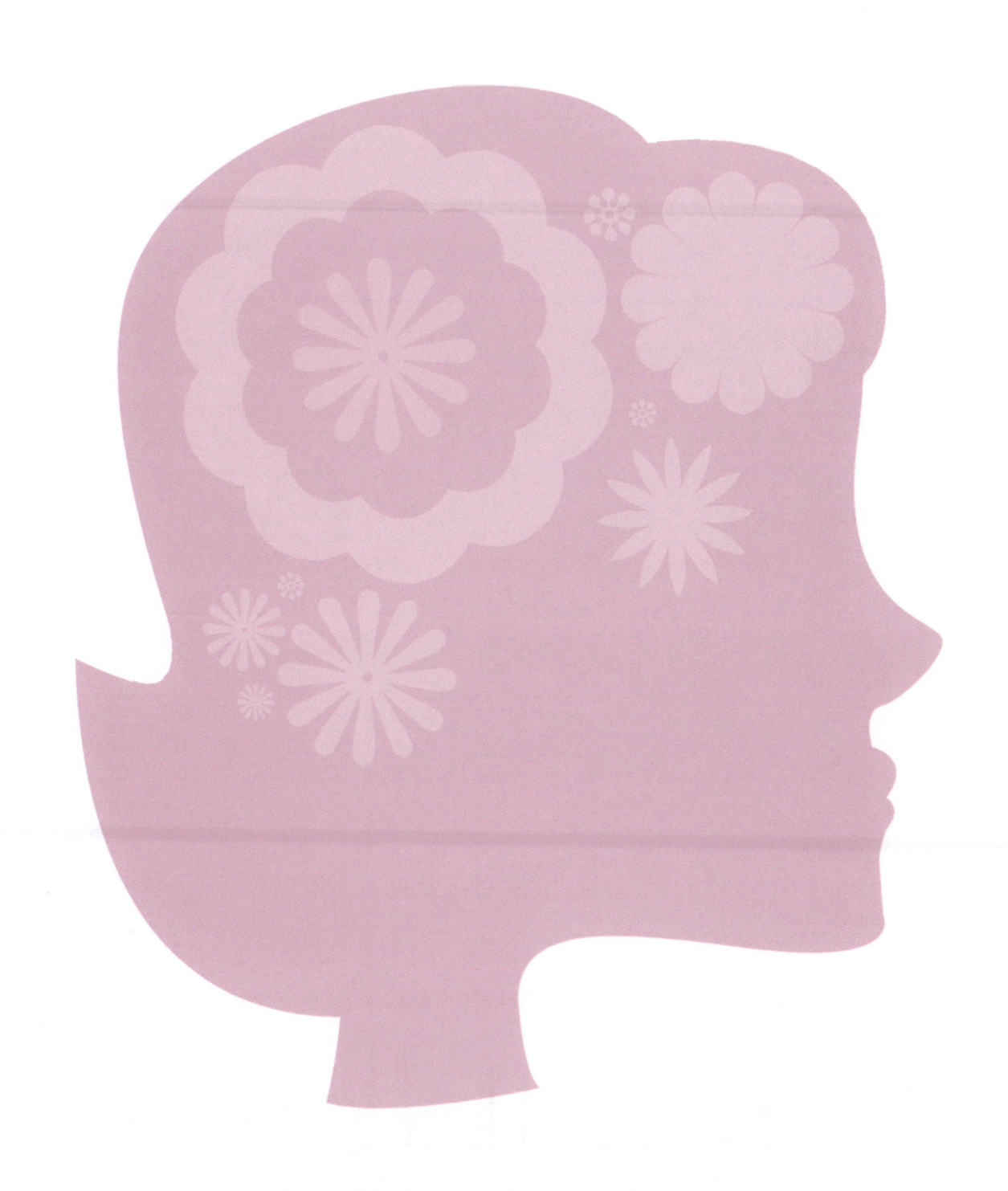

What I Eat

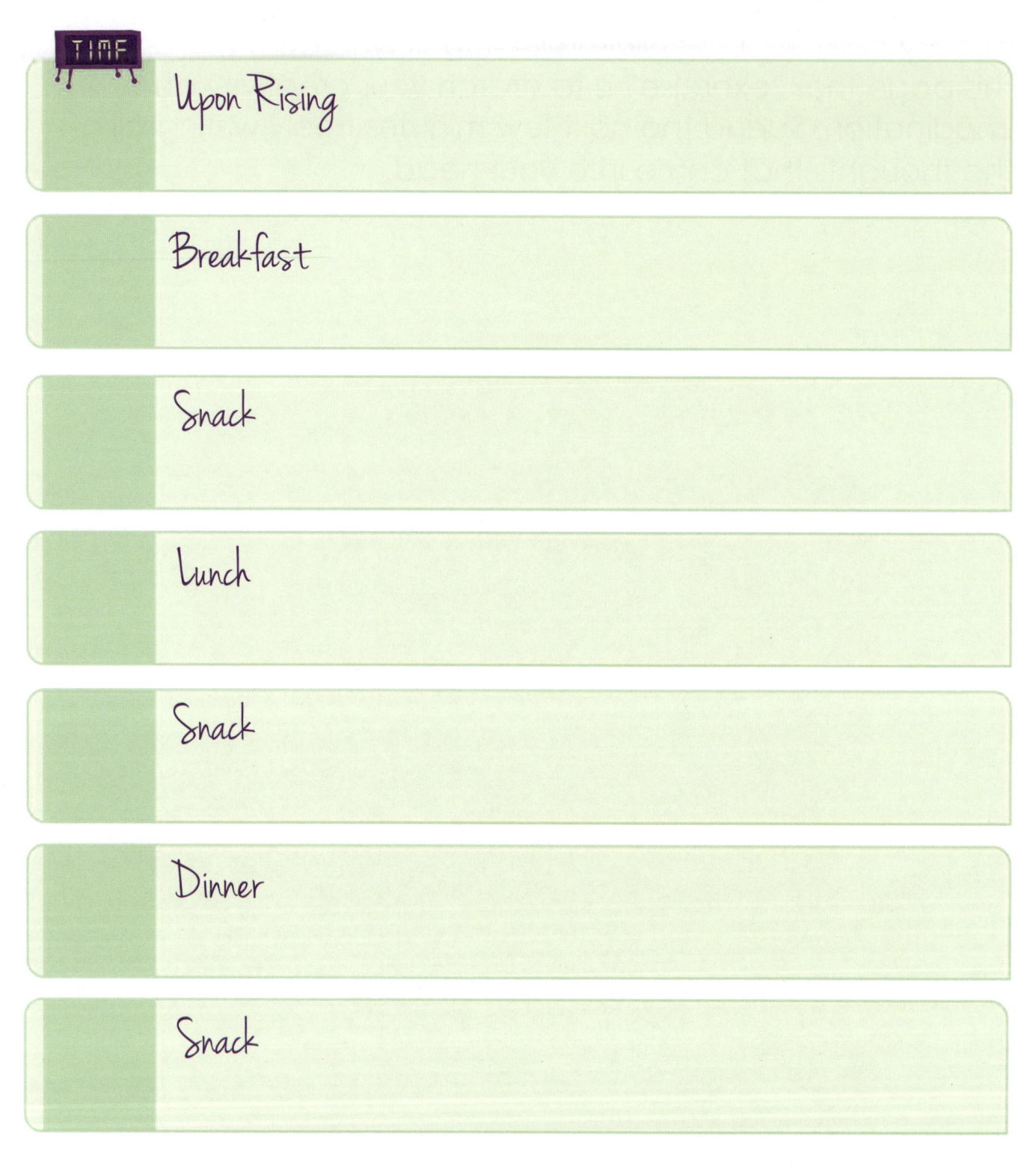

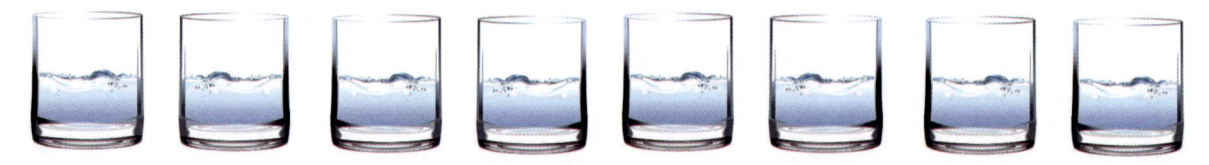

Week 2 — **Day 2**

TIME

Upon Rising

Breakfast

Snack

Lunch

Snack

Dinner

Snack

Place a check on the water cups to keep track of every 8oz you drink

Dare to Ask!

"Ask and you shall receive." When you commit your thoughts to paper, you're on your way to achieving them. Now go ahead and DARE to ask the universe for 5 things you really want... and why?

1

2

Now don't be shy...ask for what you REALLY want!

3

4

5

> **TIP**
>
> Put your best face forward. An inexpensive way to scrub your face is with oatmeal or sugar - great natural exfoliates. Then one of the best ways to tighten your pores is to rub an ice cube all over your freshly washed face - before you use your moisturizer.

What I Eat

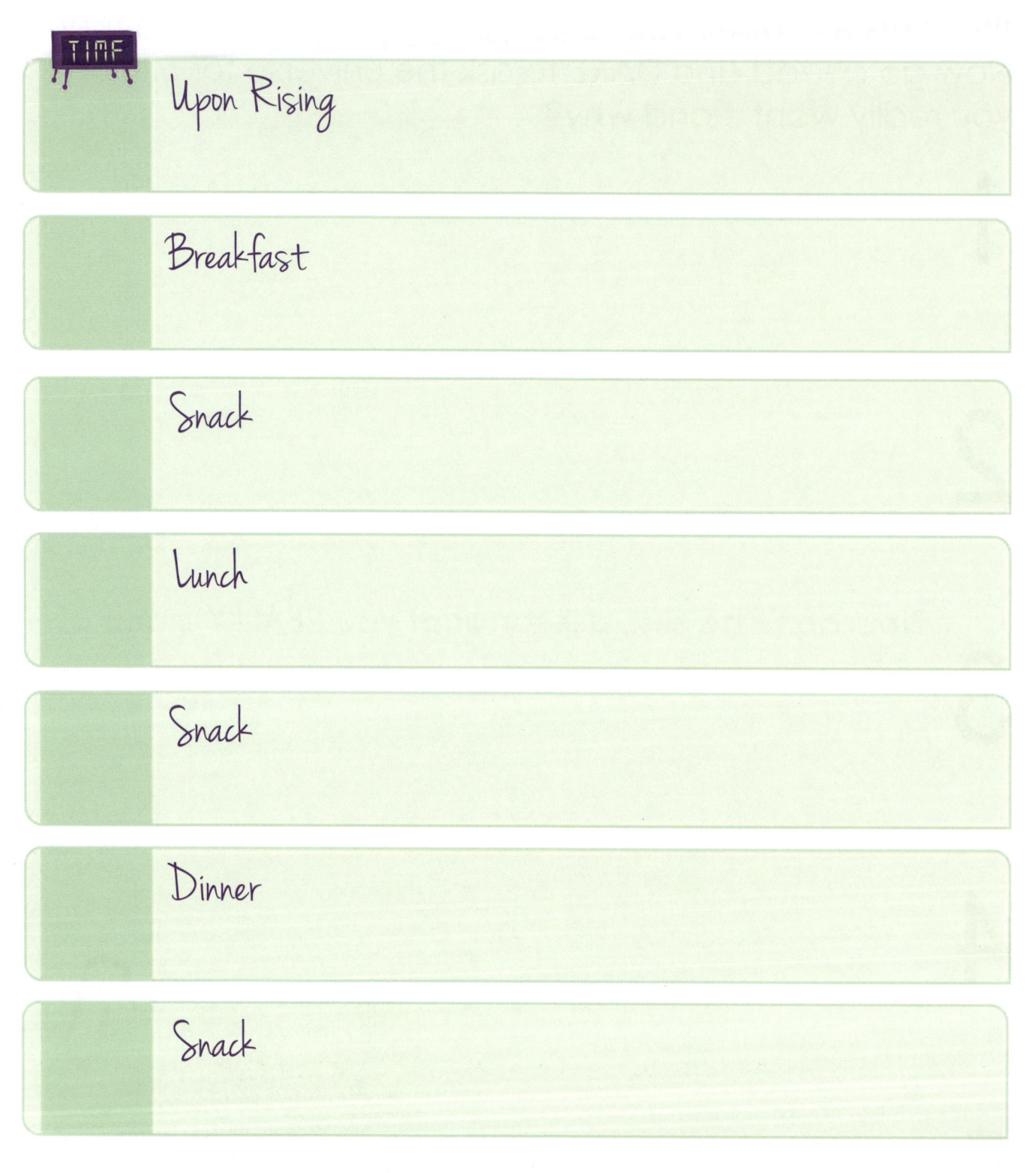

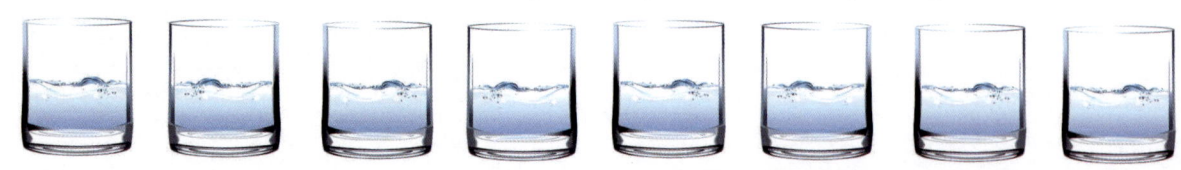

Week 2 — Day 3

TIME

- Upon Rising
- Breakfast
- Snack
- Lunch
- Snack
- Dinner
- Snack

Place a check on the water cups to keep track of every 8oz you drink

Having fun yet?

List 10 things you enjoy doing riding a bike, roller skating, romantic kissing, reading poetry, etc... When was the last time you let yourself do these things? Next to each activity write the date you last did it and the date you'd like to do it again.

1

2

3

4

5

6

7

8

9

10

xoxo

What I Eat

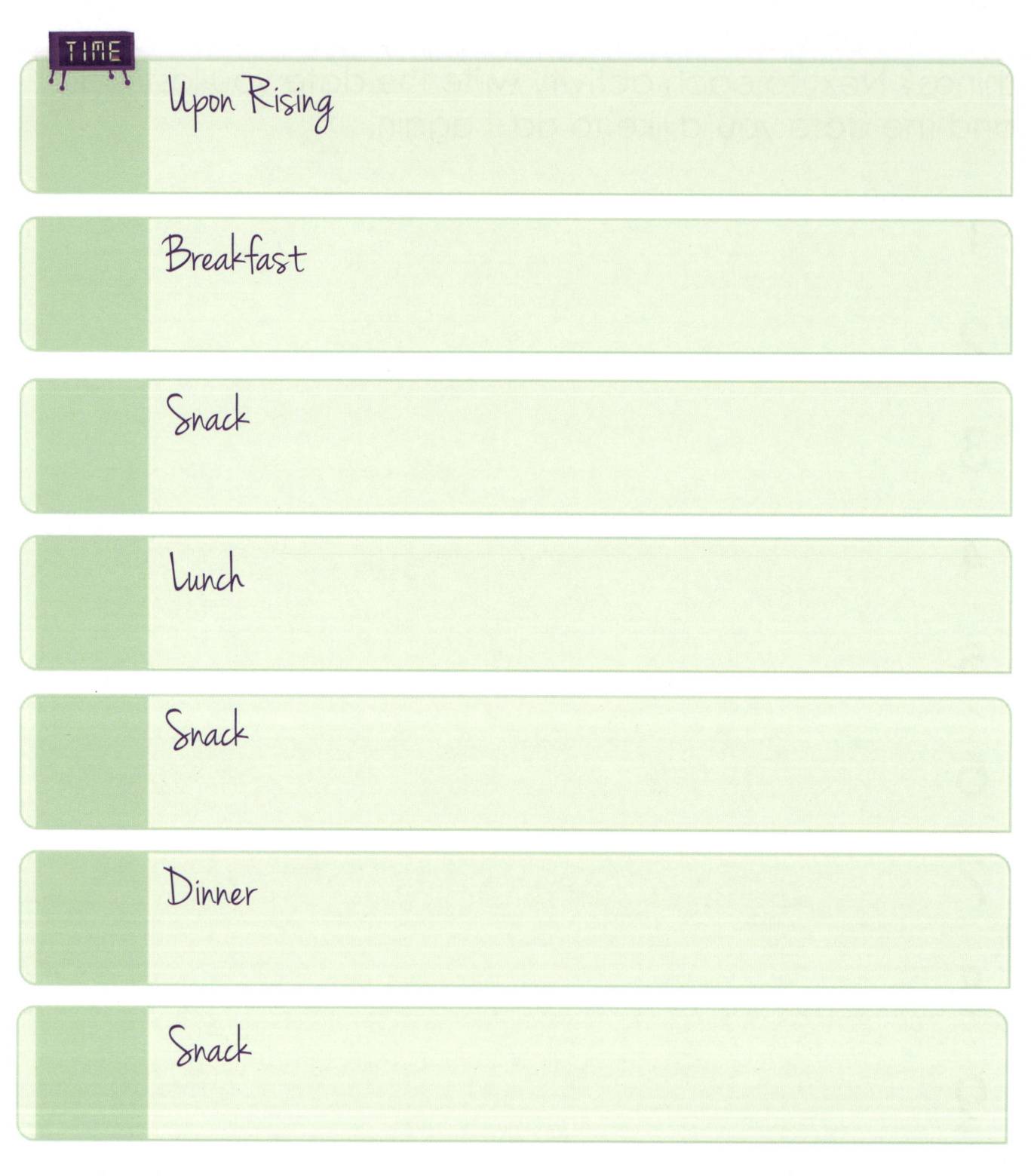

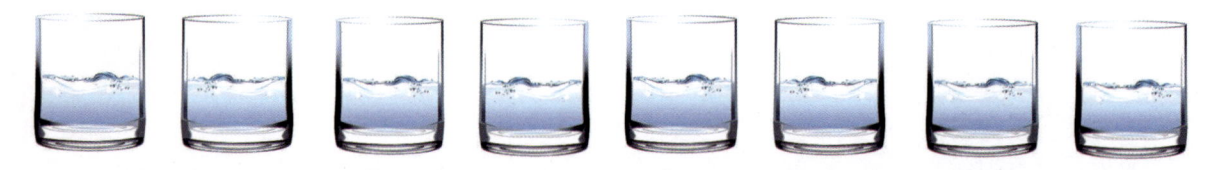

Week 2 — **Day 4**

TIME

- Upon Rising
- Breakfast
- Snack
- Lunch
- Snack
- Dinner
- Snack

Place a check on the water cups to keep track of every 8oz you drink

Shhhh... Find a quiet place to sit and write in your journal today. Make sure you're free from distractions. Now, imagine you've achieved the body you want, you're at your ideal weight. What can you do now? How do you feel?

What's different?

> **Tip**
>
> Go for a walk.
> Walking is an inexpensive way to exercise and requires no equipment other than a pair of sneakers. Note: Walking with a SpinGym gives you a great 2 for 1 workout! www.SpinGym.com.
> It's a fun and easy way to get your heart rate up into the mid-level aerobic.

Week 2 # What I Eat **Day 5**

TIME

Upon Rising

Breakfast

Snack

Lunch

Snack

Dinner

Snack

Place a check on the water cups to keep track of every 8oz you drink

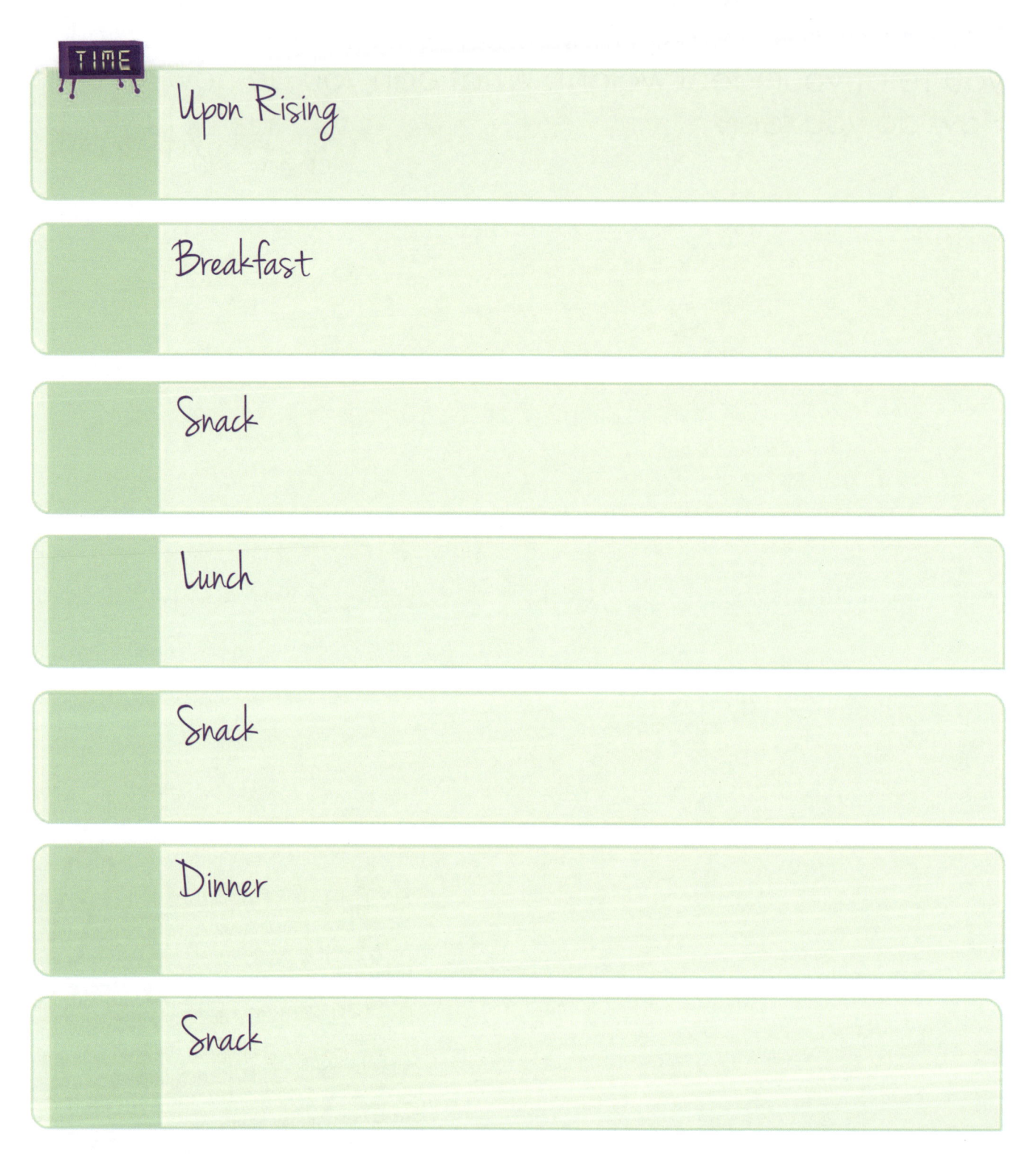

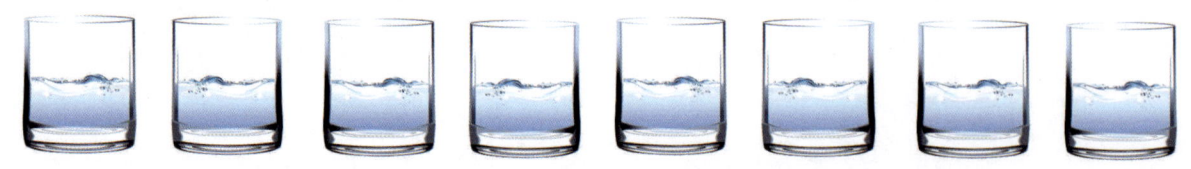

46

The power of small steps and tiny changes.

List 10 changes you would like to make for yourself, from big to little. For example: explore a new hairstyle, join a gym, get a pet, paint the kitchen, buy new furniture, replace old towels...

1
2
3
4
5
6
7
8
9
10

TIP
Choose one of the changes above... and actually do it TODAY!

What I Eat

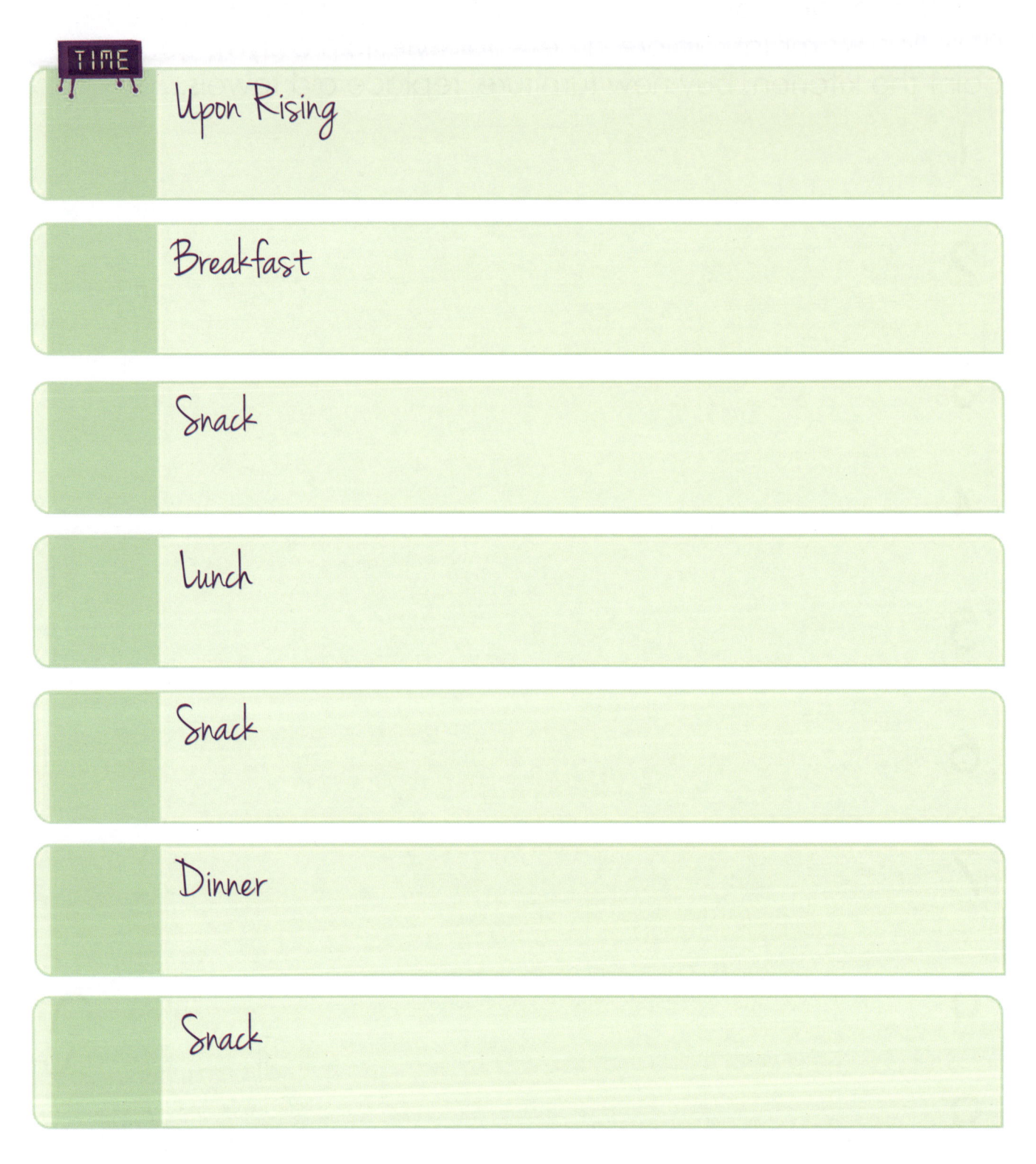

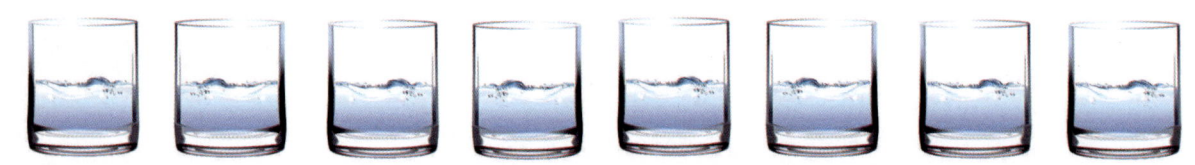

Week 2 — **Day 6**

TIME

- Upon Rising
- Breakfast
- Snack
- Lunch
- Snack
- Dinner
- Snack

Place a check on the water cups to keep track of every 8oz you drink

Role models are important. List 3 people you admire (whether you know them or not). What traits do you admire and how can you create and develop those traits in yourself?

1

2

3

Tip

Hungry? Sometimes the brain confuses thirst for hunger. So drink a glass of water. For fun, add a slice of lemon or a packet of a no-calorie powdered beverage mix. It's important to get your 6-8 glasses everyday! If you're still hungry 15 minutes later, THEN eat.

What I Eat

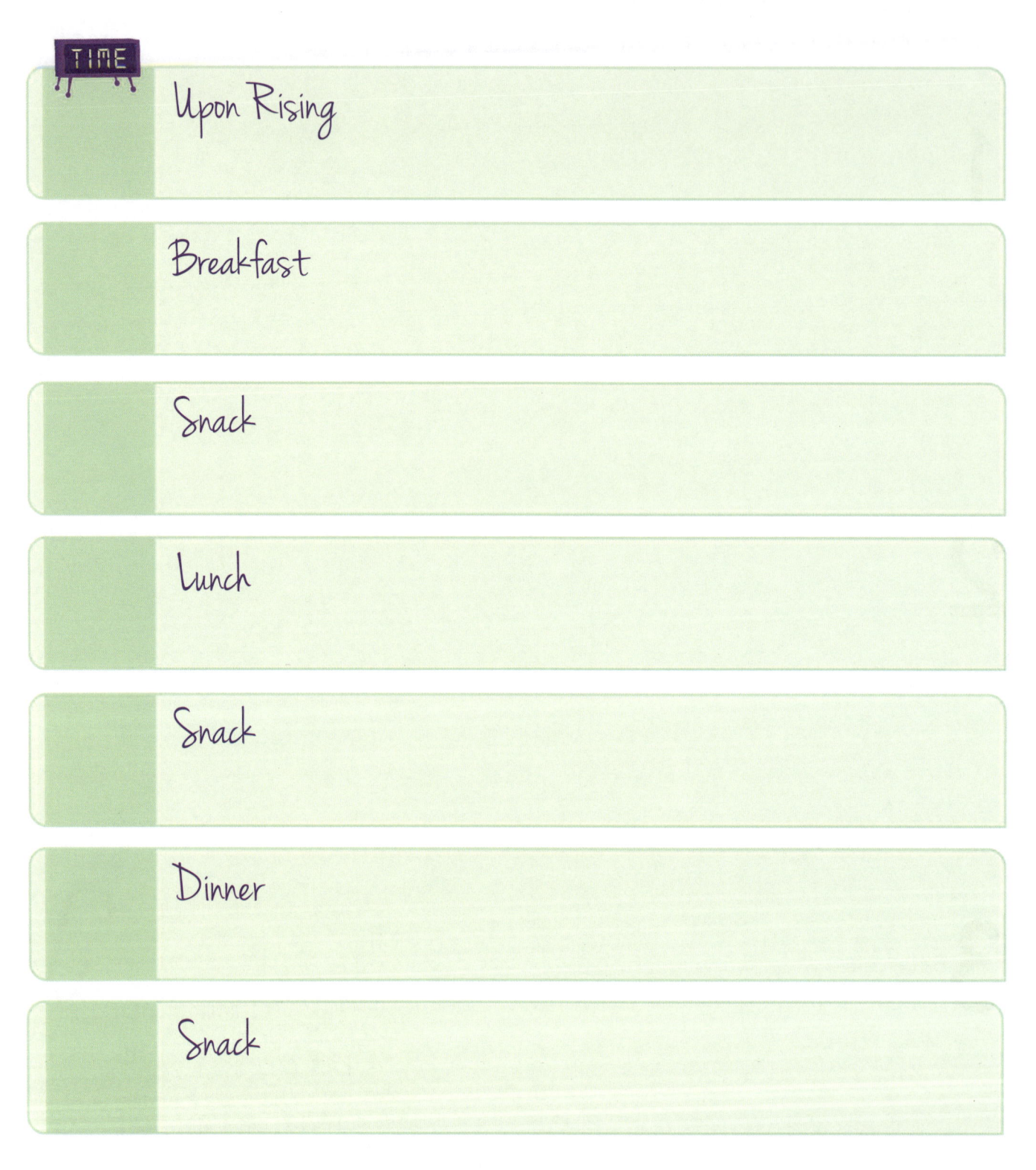

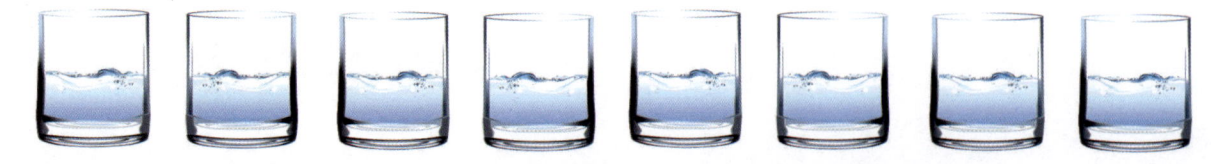

Week 2 **Day 7**

TIME

Upon Rising

Breakfast

Snack

Lunch

Snack

Dinner

Snack

Place a check on the water cups to keep track of every 8oz you drink

Congrats! You have made it to the end of the 2nd week. Time to check in with yourself.

1 How many days this week did you fill in your journal? Write the number, not the excuses.

> Fill in the number of days
> *be honest!*

2 Biggest obstacles this week:
List strategies for overcoming them.

3 What are your goals for the future?

The Joy of Juicing

A great snack idea is a 6-8 oz. glass of fresh squeezed juice. *Nothing in a can, carton, or juice box!* All ingredients should be raw and organic when possible. Since 2003, I have had the honor of co-hosting the Power Juicer infomercial with the legendary fitness guru Jack LaLanne and his wife Elaine. They have helped me and millions of people around the world understand the nutritional benefits of fresh squeezed juices. We juiced everything from apples, carrots and celery to sweet potato, beets and broccoli. I have included some of my favorite juicing recipes on the next page. Don't forget the pulp from juicing is great to add to muffins, carrot cake and soups. My recommendation is to purchase a high speed, wide mouthed, quality juicer, like Jack LaLanne's. (Hint, hint...)

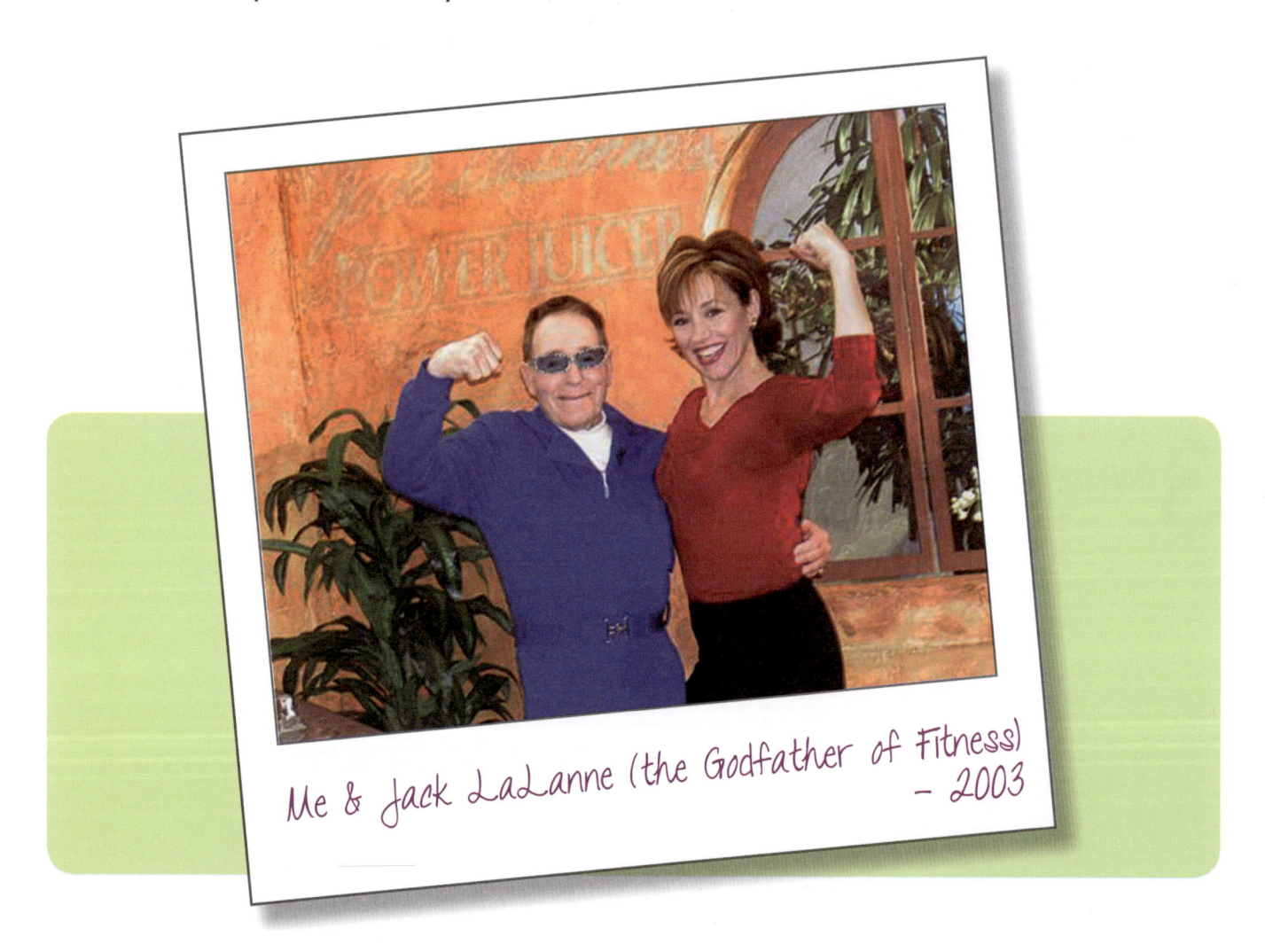

Me & Jack LaLanne (the Godfather of Fitness) - 2003

My Favorite Juicing Recipes

No Need for Reading Glasses, Carrot Juice!
6 carrots, 2 stalks of celery, 1/2 beet, 1 apple

Pineapple Pick-Me-Up
4 slices of pineapple, 4-6 large strawberries, 1 bunch red grapes, 1/2 peeled orange

Berry Blitz
1 cup blueberries, 1 cup strawberries, 1 peach, 1 apple, 1/2 lb red seedless grapes

"Sleeveless in 6" - Green Supreme
1/2 cup broccoli, 1/2 cup spinach, 3 celery stalks, 1 cucumber, 4 medium carrots, 1 green apple.
(For added zest, add 2 slices peeled ginger)

The Forbes Riley Fizz
1 ripe mango, 4 pineapple spears, 2 kiwi fruit, 6 strawberries, 1 large carrot, 4 oz sparkling mineral water or champagne

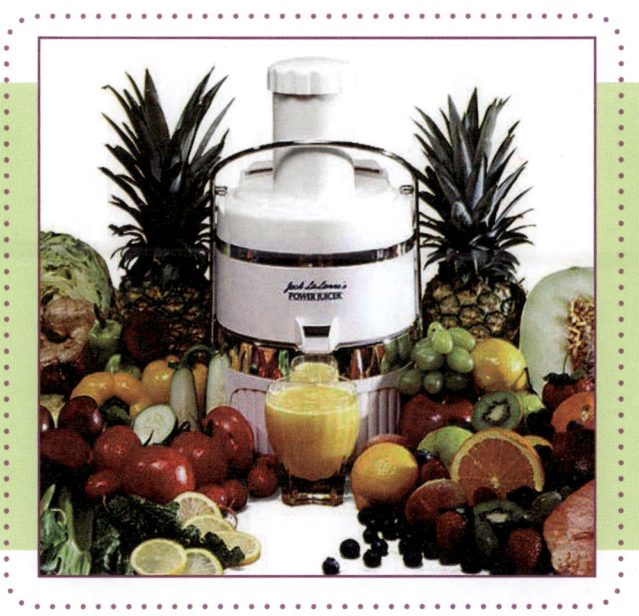

Calcium as we know comes from dairy products, but a variety of vegetables also provide substantial calcium - try adding any one of these to your juicing recipes: broccoli, collard greens, kale, kohlrabi, okra, or turnip greens.

Fun and Healthy e.a.t. Recipe #2

Ben Franklin Parchment Protein

Fish is a great nutritious source of protein. Here is a list of my favorites:

Alaska Wild Salmon	Atlantic Char	Clams (steamers)
Cod	Halibut	Grouper
Mahi-mahi	Mussels	Orange Roughy
Pollack	Rainbow Trout	Red Snapper
Scallops	Shrimp	Swordfish
Tilapia	Trout	Tuna

Try to avoid fried fish, as it adds unwanted calories and oil. Fish is great baked, broiled or grilled. Here's a creative way to serve and eat fish... in parchment paper!

Here ye, Here ye -- Something's Fishy!!

Ingredients

4 (4 oz) fillets of cod/tilapia/salmon, rinsed and patted dry

2 tbsp extra-virgin olive oil

1/2 tsp salt

1/2 tsp pepper

4-6 oz mixed mushrooms (sliced portabello, shiitake, button)

1 bag of pre-cleaned baby spinach

4 tbsp lemon zest

4 tbsp shredded fresh basil

1 glove garlic, diced

1/2 cup sliced red onion

Directions

1. Preheat the oven to 425°F. Prepare 4 sheets of parchment paper (approx 16" square) Have 2 baking sheets ready.

2. Fold the parchment squares in 1/2, forming 2 rectangles. Close to the fold on each piece place the fish fillet. Drizzle with 1/2 tsp of olive oil and sprinkle with salt and pepper. Scatter the mushrooms, spinach, lemon zest, basil and onion on top. Repeat with all 4 fillets on their own parchment.

3. Fold the parchment across the fish and then fold the edges to create an airtight packet. Place the fish parchment packets on the baking sheet and place in the oven. Bake until the paper puffs up and the fish gives when pressed through the packet. Approx 10 minutes

Delicious, nutritious, unique and easy to prepare.

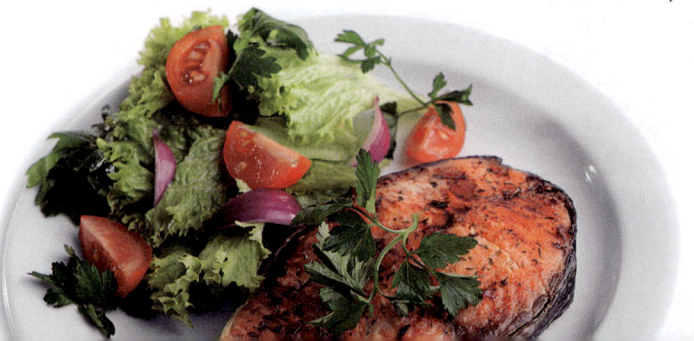

Bon Appetit!

Forbes Fit & Fun

Wordsearch is one of my favorite distractions. I have included it in this book so you can kill time in a creative and fun way. Hidden in the grid of letters are inspiring words. They can be forward, backwards, up, down, or diagonal. When you find the word, take a moment and see how it affects your life.

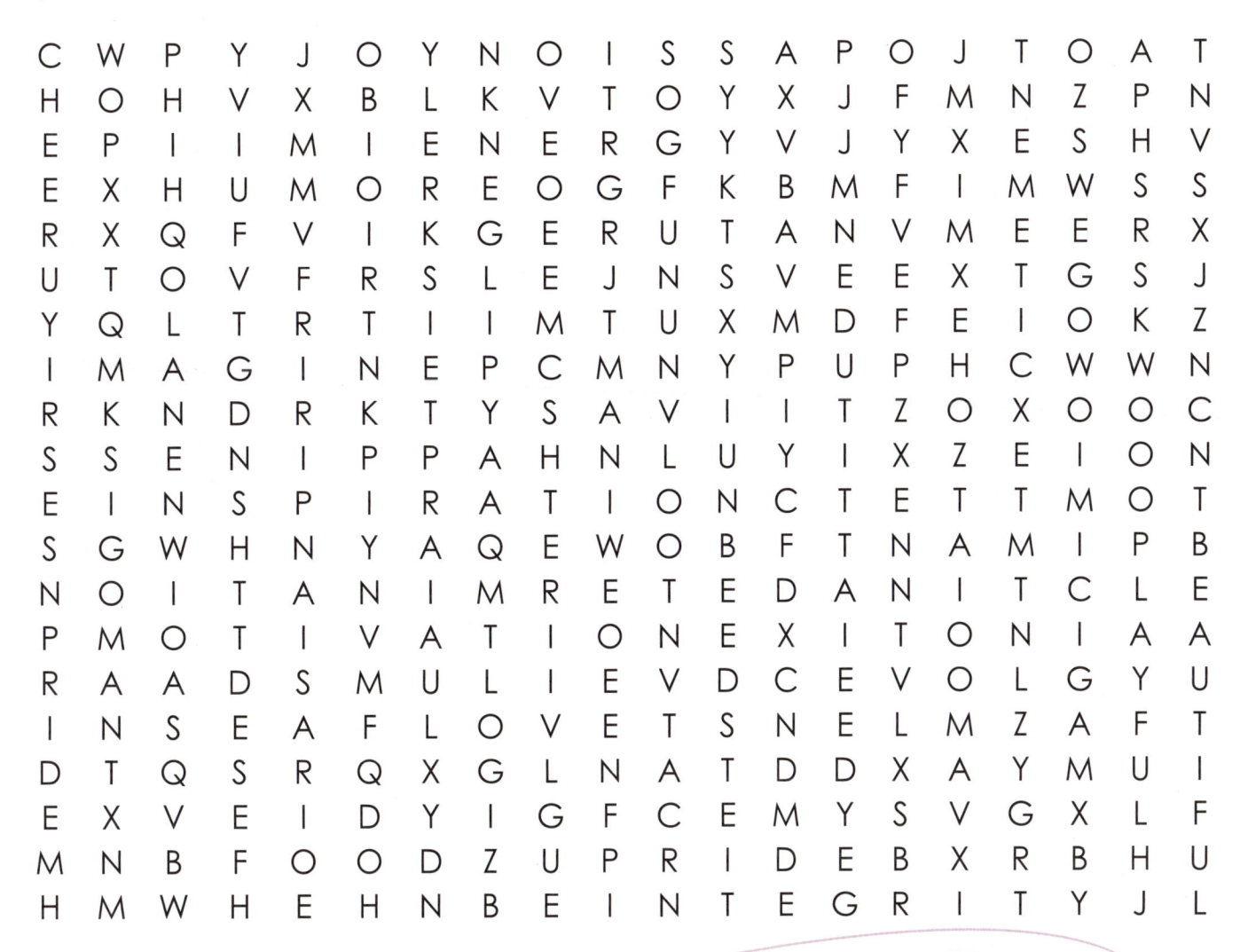

```
C W P Y J O Y N O I S S A P O J T O A T
H O H V X B L K V T O Y X J F M N Z P N
E P I I M I E N E R G Y V J Y X E S H V
E X H U M O R E O G F K B M F I M W S S
R X Q F V I K G E R U T A N V M E E R X
U T O V F R S L E J N S V E E X T G S J
Y Q L T R T I I M T U X M D F E I O K Z
I M A G I N E P C M N Y P U P H C W W N
R K N D R K T Y S A V I I T Z O X O O C
S S E N I P P A H N L U Y I X Z E I O N
E I N S P I R A T I O N C T E T T M O T
S G W H N Y A Q E W O B F T N A M I P B
N O I T A N I M R E T E D A N I T C L E
P M O T I V A T I O N E X I T O N I A A
R A A D S M U L I E V D C E V O L G Y U
I N S E A F L O V E T S N E L M Z A F T
D T Q S R Q X G L N A T D D X A Y M U I
E X V E I D Y I G F C E M Y S V G X L F
M N B F O O D Z U P R I D E B X R B H U
H M W H E H N B E I N T E G R I T Y J L
```

	Excitement	Joy
Attitude	Fascination	Love
Beautiful	Food	Magic
Cheer	Fun	Motivation
Commitment	Happiness	Nature
Determination	Imagine	Passion
Devotion	Inspiration	Playful
Dream	Integrity	Pride
Energy	Joy	Whimsical

Notes

"Without goals, and plans to reach them, you are like a ship that has set sail with no destination."

— Fitzhugh Dodson

Week 3

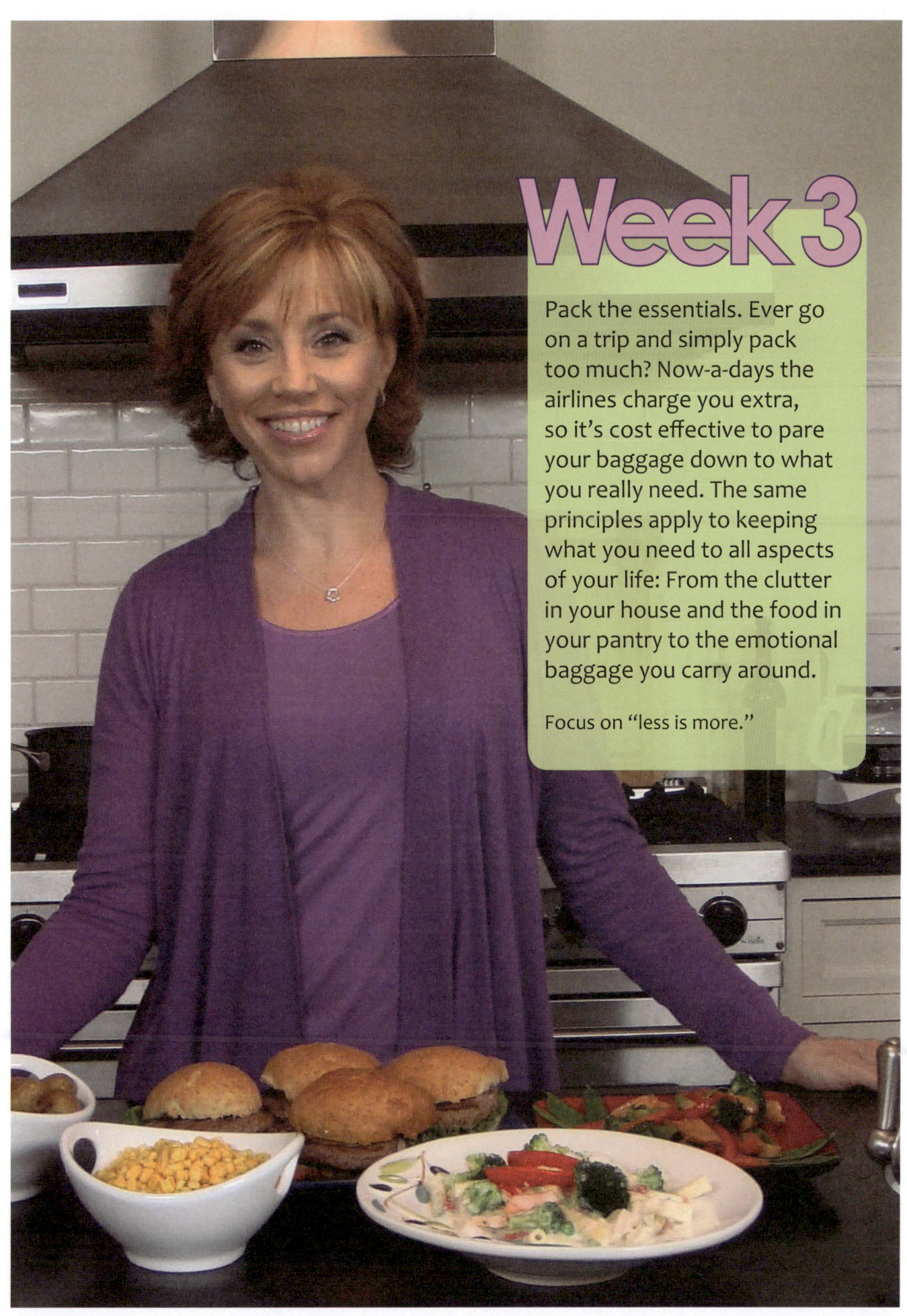

Pack the essentials. Ever go on a trip and simply pack too much? Now-a-days the airlines charge you extra, so it's cost effective to pare your baggage down to what you really need. The same principles apply to keeping what you need to all aspects of your life: From the clutter in your house and the food in your pantry to the emotional baggage you carry around.

Focus on "less is more."

Week 3 # What I Eat **Day 1**

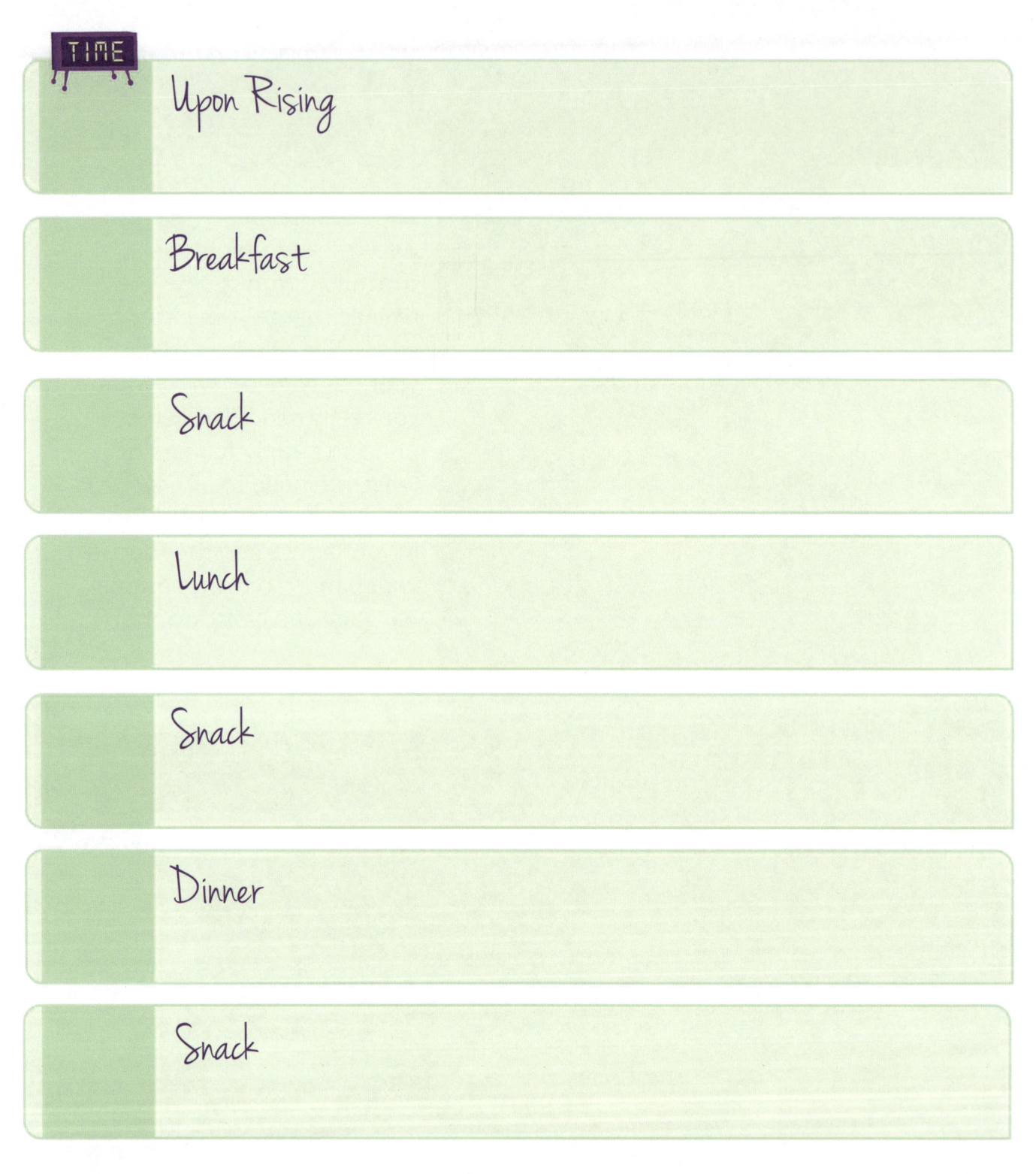

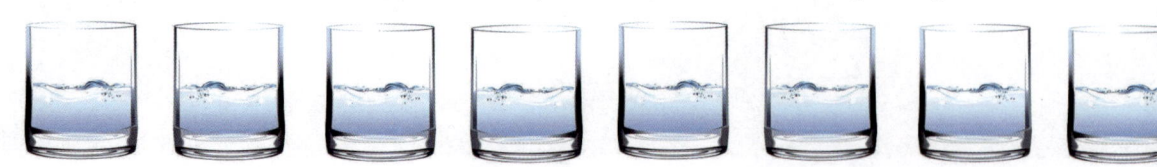

TIME

Upon Rising

Breakfast

Snack

Lunch

Snack

Dinner

Snack

Place a check on the water cups to keep track of every 8oz you drink

Let's have some fun. Spend a few minutes today dreaming about what a perfect dinner party would be like.

1 Who would you invite? (perhaps famous, living or dead)

2 What part of the world is this amazing dinner taking place?

3 Write about some of the foods you will be serving.

4 Rate your evening on a scale of 1 to 10.

What I Eat

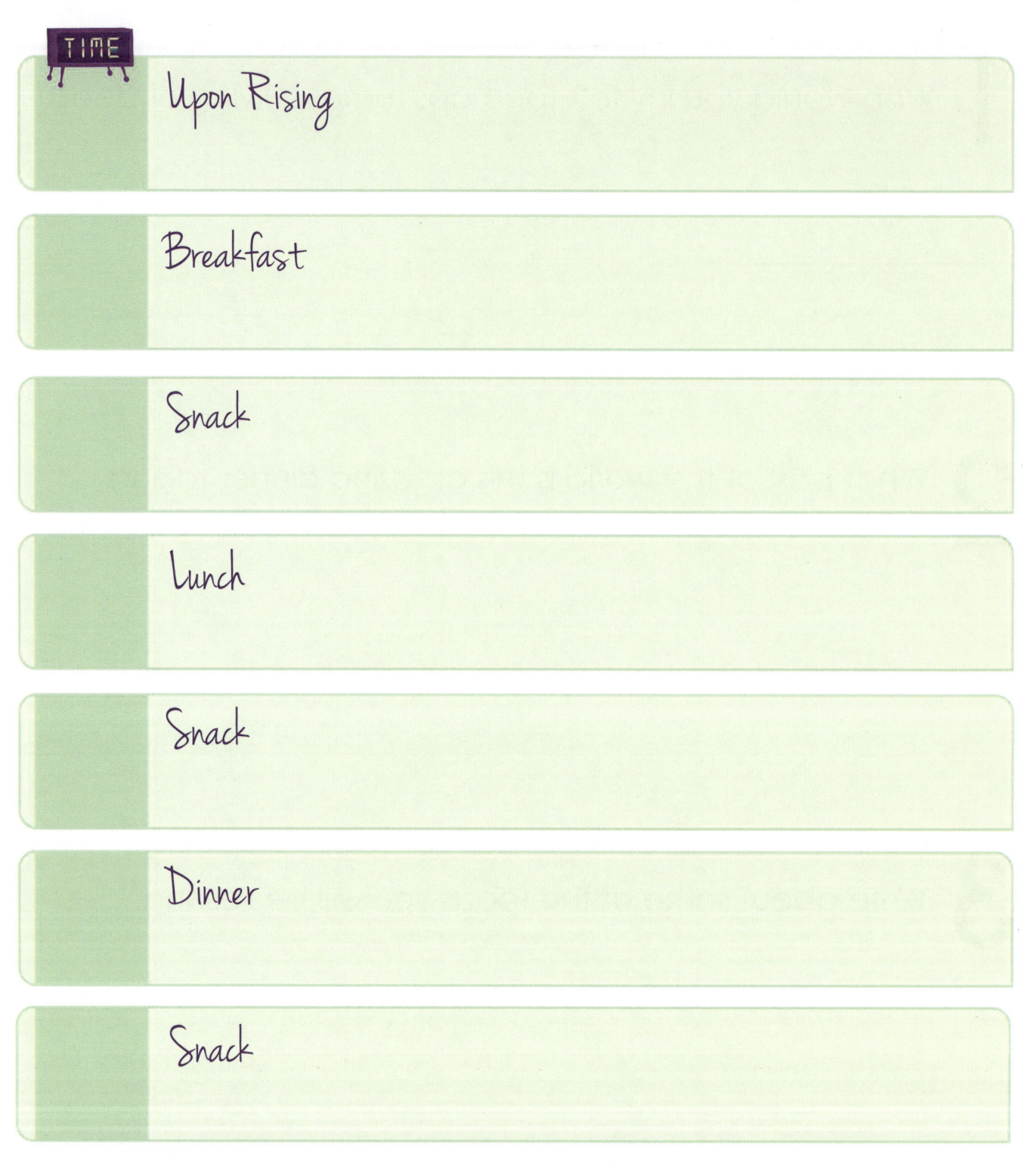

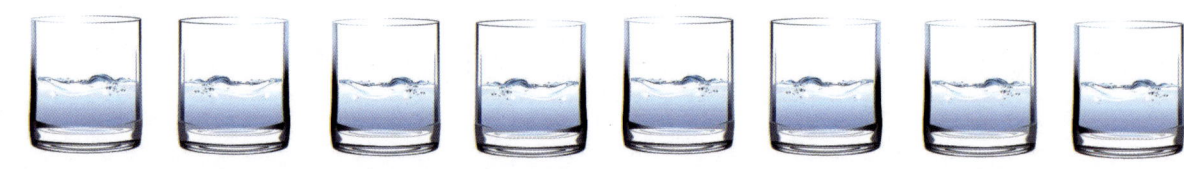

Week 3 — **Day 2**

TIME

- Upon Rising
- Breakfast
- Snack
- Lunch
- Snack
- Dinner
- Snack

Place a check on the water cups to keep track of every 8oz you drink

Imagine

3 "out of character" things you've thought of doing, but haven't. For example; skydiving, belly dancing, buying a drum set, pole dancing, taking an art class.
Now draw a picture of yourself doing one of them!

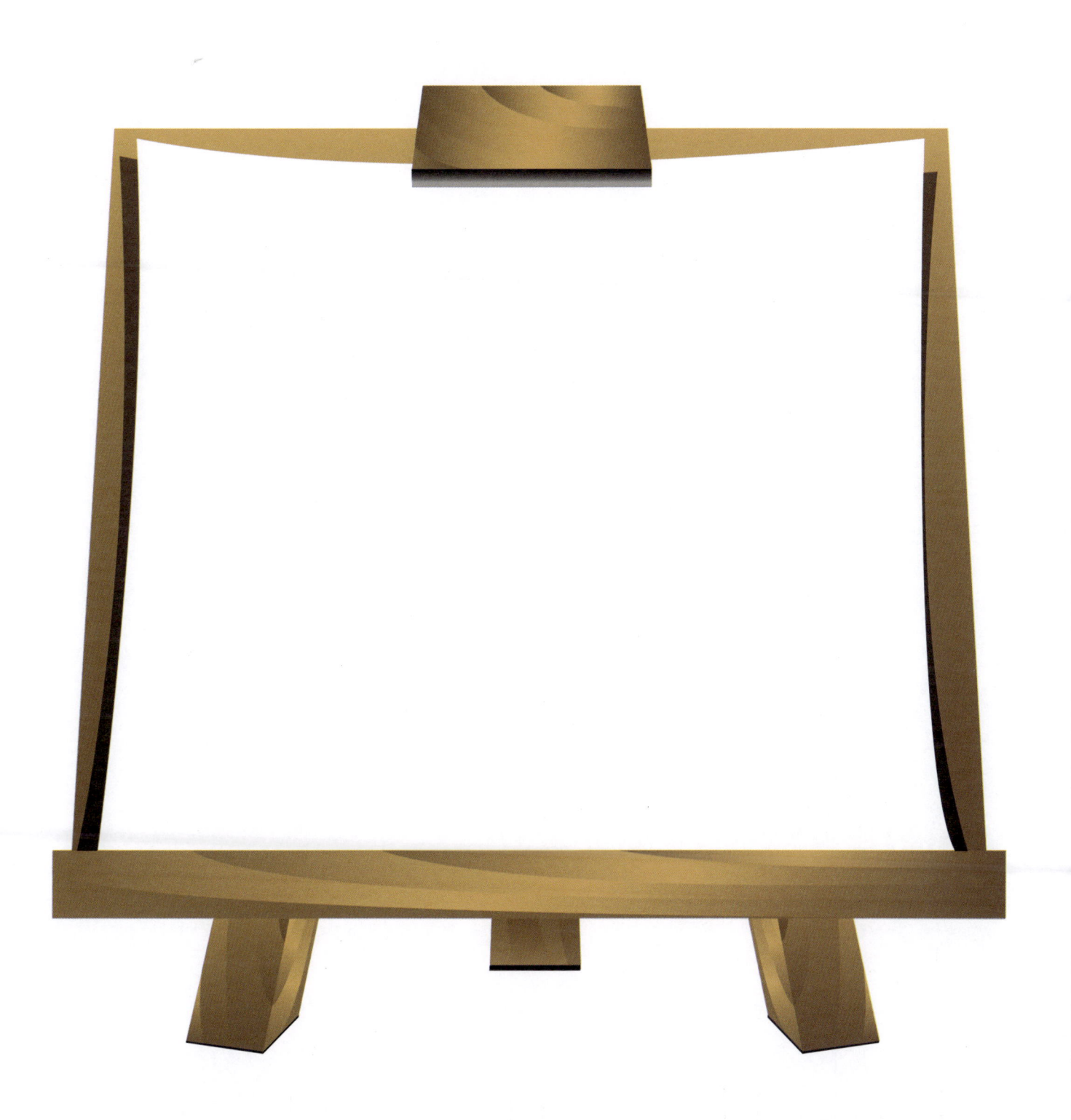

What I Eat

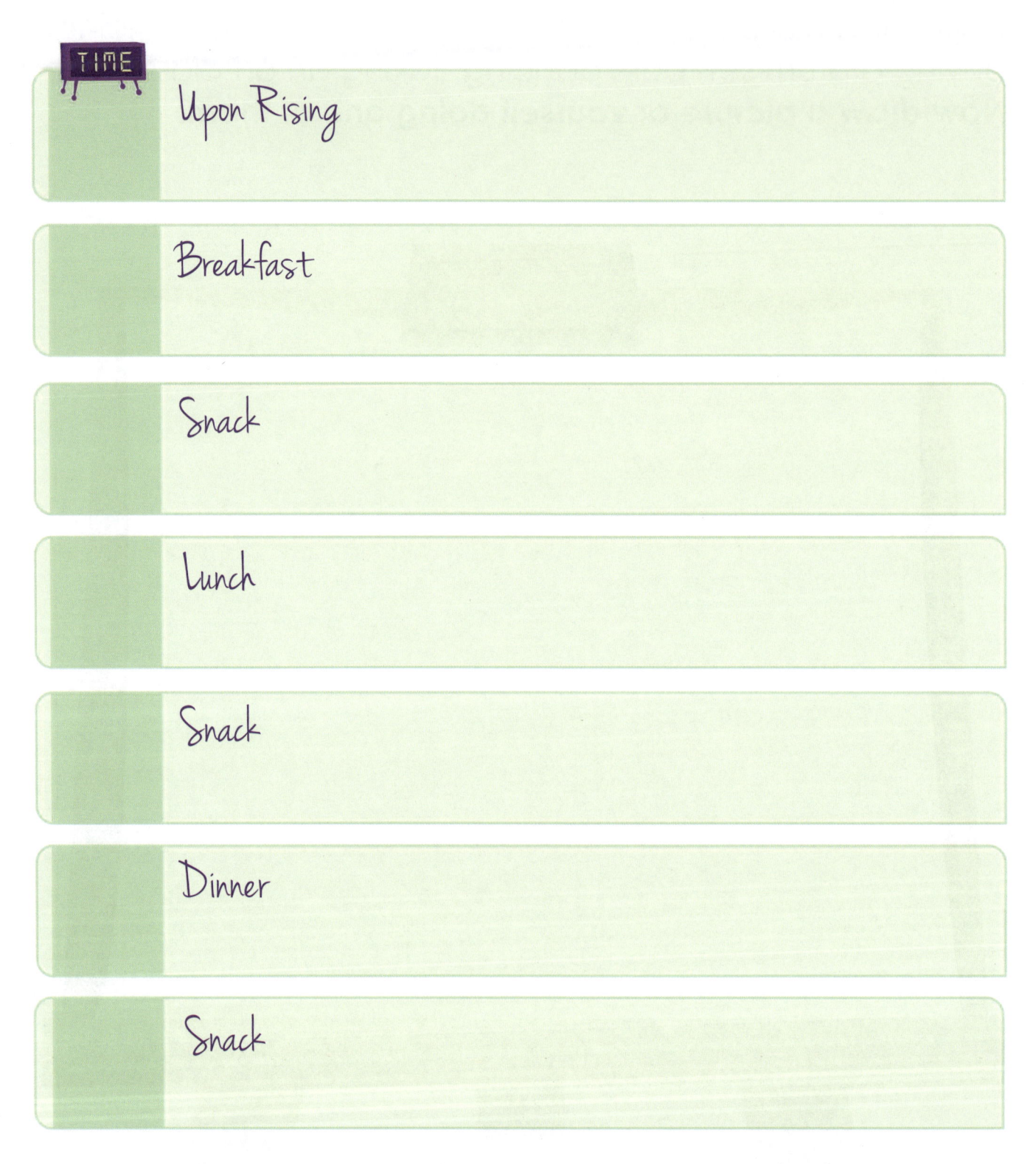

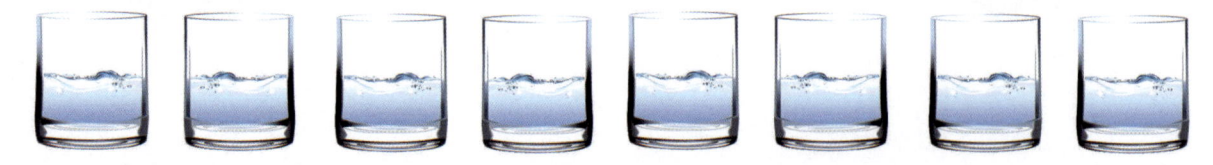

Week 3 — **Day 3**

TIME

- Upon Rising
- Breakfast
- Snack
- Lunch
- Snack
- Dinner
- Snack

Place a check on the water cups to keep track of every 8oz you drink

Write an *imaginary story* to a child explaining how an animal came to be. For example: Why does a zebra have stripes? Why does a giraffe have a long neck? Why does a snake have no legs?

Be Creative Fill this entire page with the story!

> **TIP**
>
> Go to the zoo and observe the animals. Watch how animals eat the same meal every day and never ask for dessert.
>
> Lions eat meat, giraffes eat leaves, and elephants eat grass. Stop and ponder about what you eat daily... and when

What I Eat

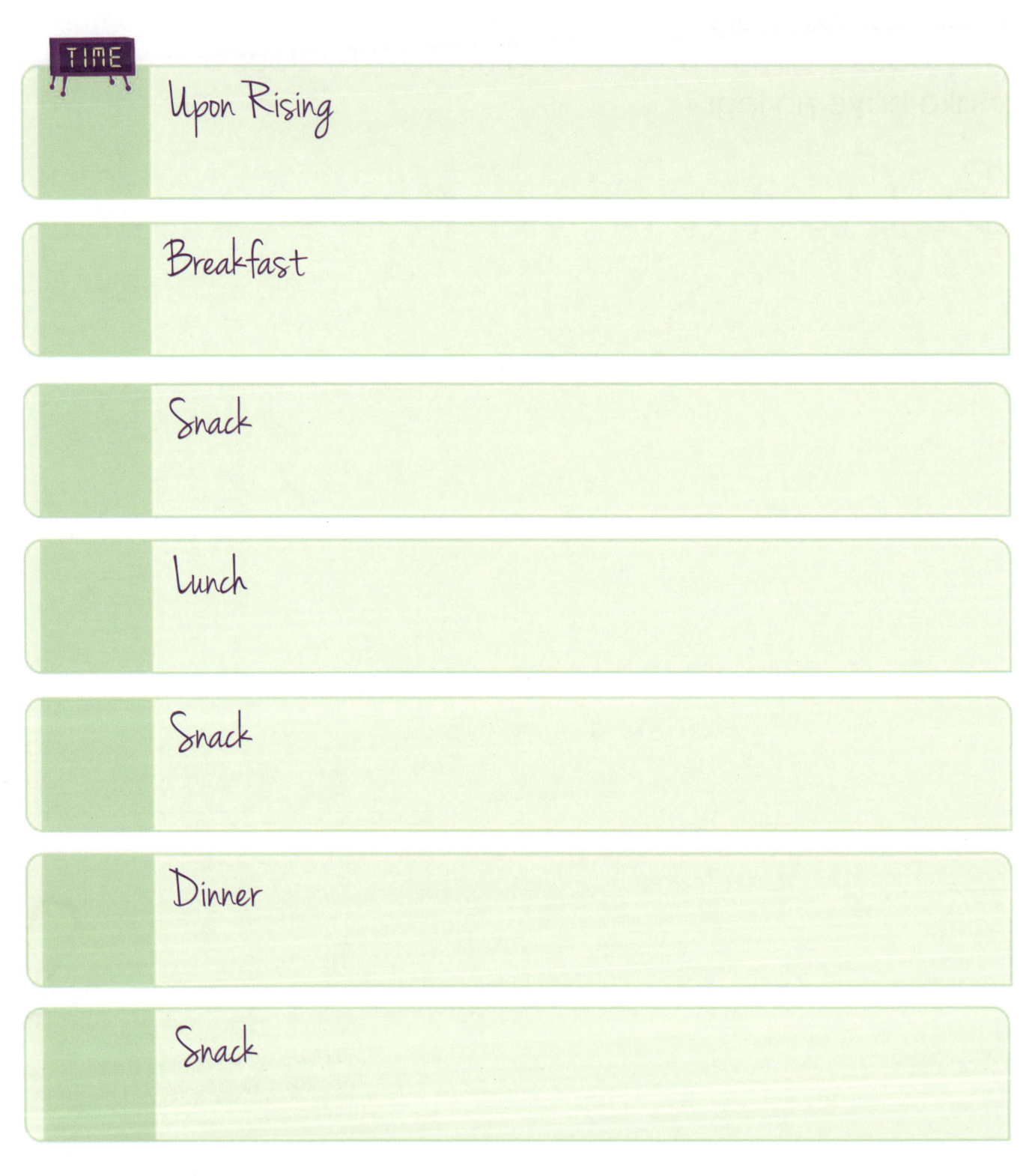

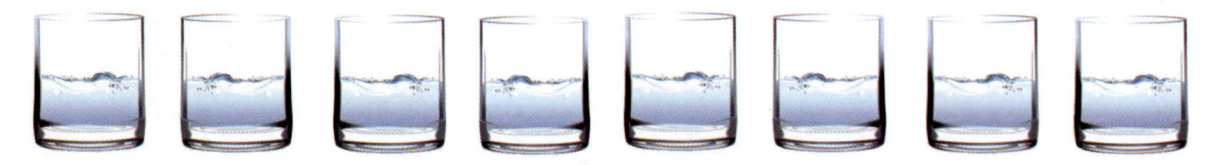

Week 3 — Day 4

TIME

Upon Rising

Breakfast

Snack

Lunch

Snack

Dinner

Snack

Place a check on the water cups to keep track of every 8oz you drink

Fill in the blanks!

I remember the time when:

I feel guilty when I:

My biggest joy in life is:

If all of my dreams came true I would:

Tip

Peanut butter & jelly sandwiches can remind you of being a kid. On whole wheat bread or Wasa crackers, PB+J can be a nutritious snack. Make sure you choose an organic, natural peanut butter with no sugar and a healthy no-cal fruit spread.

… Week 3 … **What I Eat** … Day 5

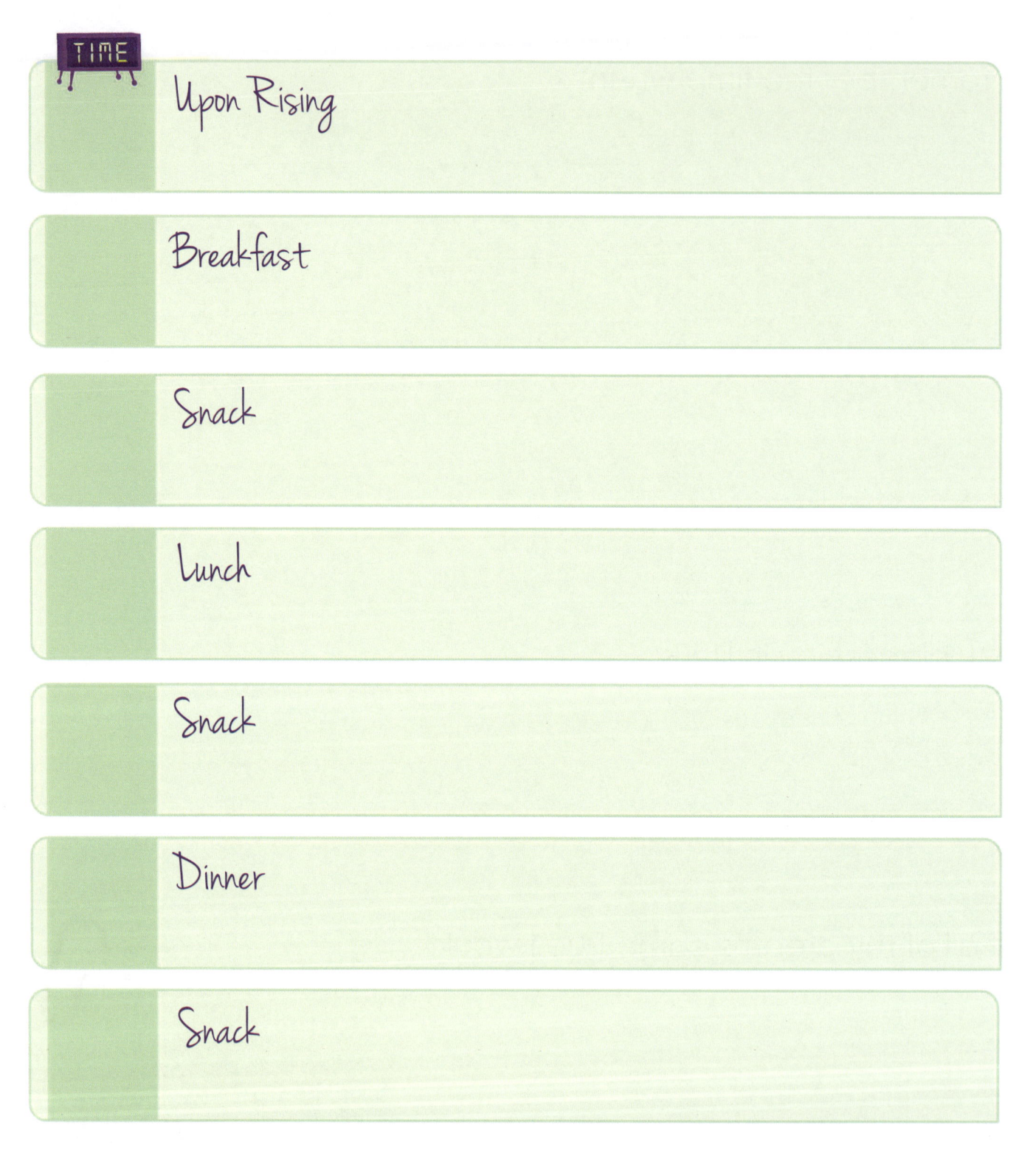

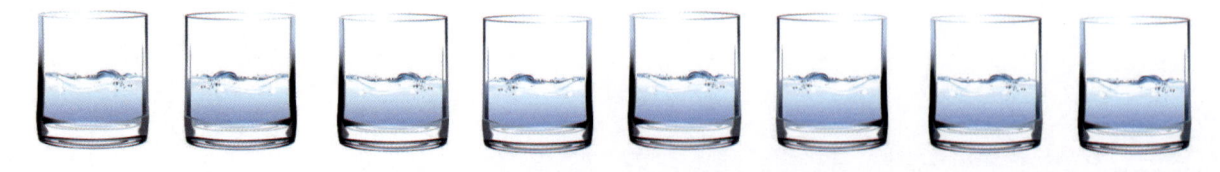

TIME

Upon Rising

Breakfast

Snack

Lunch

Snack

Dinner

Snack

Place a check on the water cups to keep track of every 8oz you drink

Abundance (uh-buhn-duh-ns) noun

1. An extremely plentiful supply or quantity
2. Unlimited supply; overflowing fullness (abundance of joy, love & happiness)

Fill in each of the areas below with your definition of abundance.

Family:

Health:

Wealth:

> **TIP**
>
> Take a bath. Novels romanticize them, but nothing is quite as luxurious as a warm soak. Include some fragrant bath or Epsom salts, a few candles and some music.
>
> Relax.

What I Eat

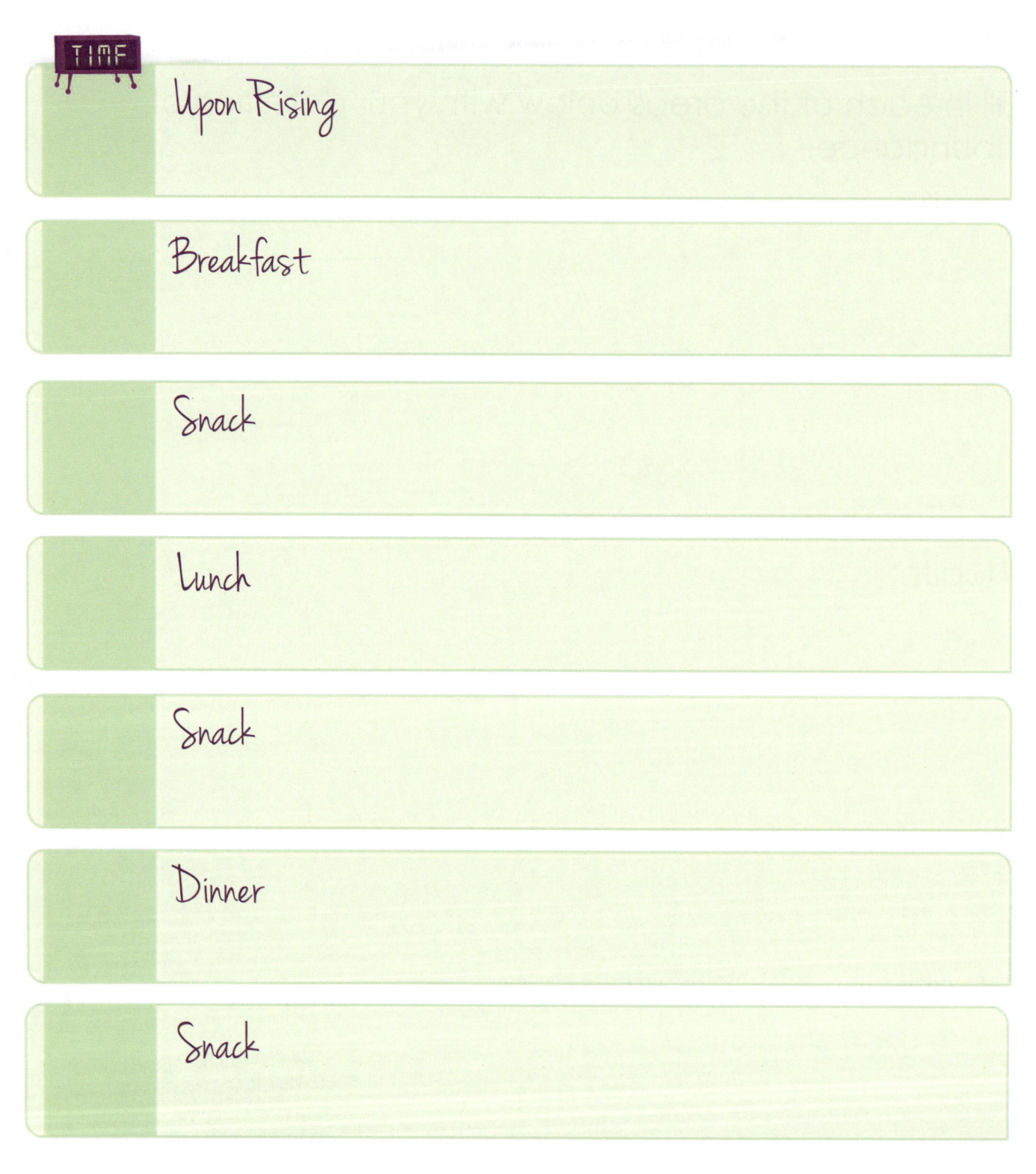

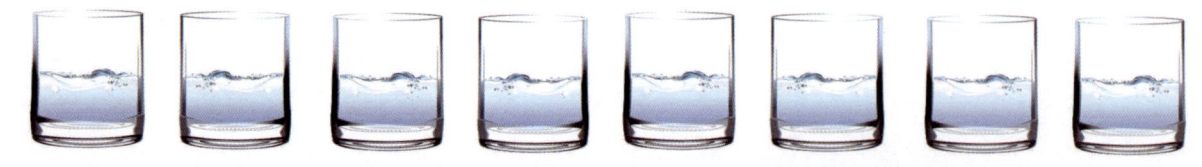

Week 3 — **Day 6**

TIME

- Upon Rising
- Breakfast
- Snack
- Lunch
- Snack
- Dinner
- Snack

Place a check on the water cups to keep track of every 8oz you drink

They say, "Money makes the world go round."
What does money mean to you?

Money means:

In my family money represented:

Not having money is:

If I had more money, I would:

TIP

Don't be afraid of your waiter. When eating out, encourage your server to help you stay on target. Ask for sauces & salad dressing on the side, substitute a veggie for the potato and replace fried meats with grilled.

What I Eat

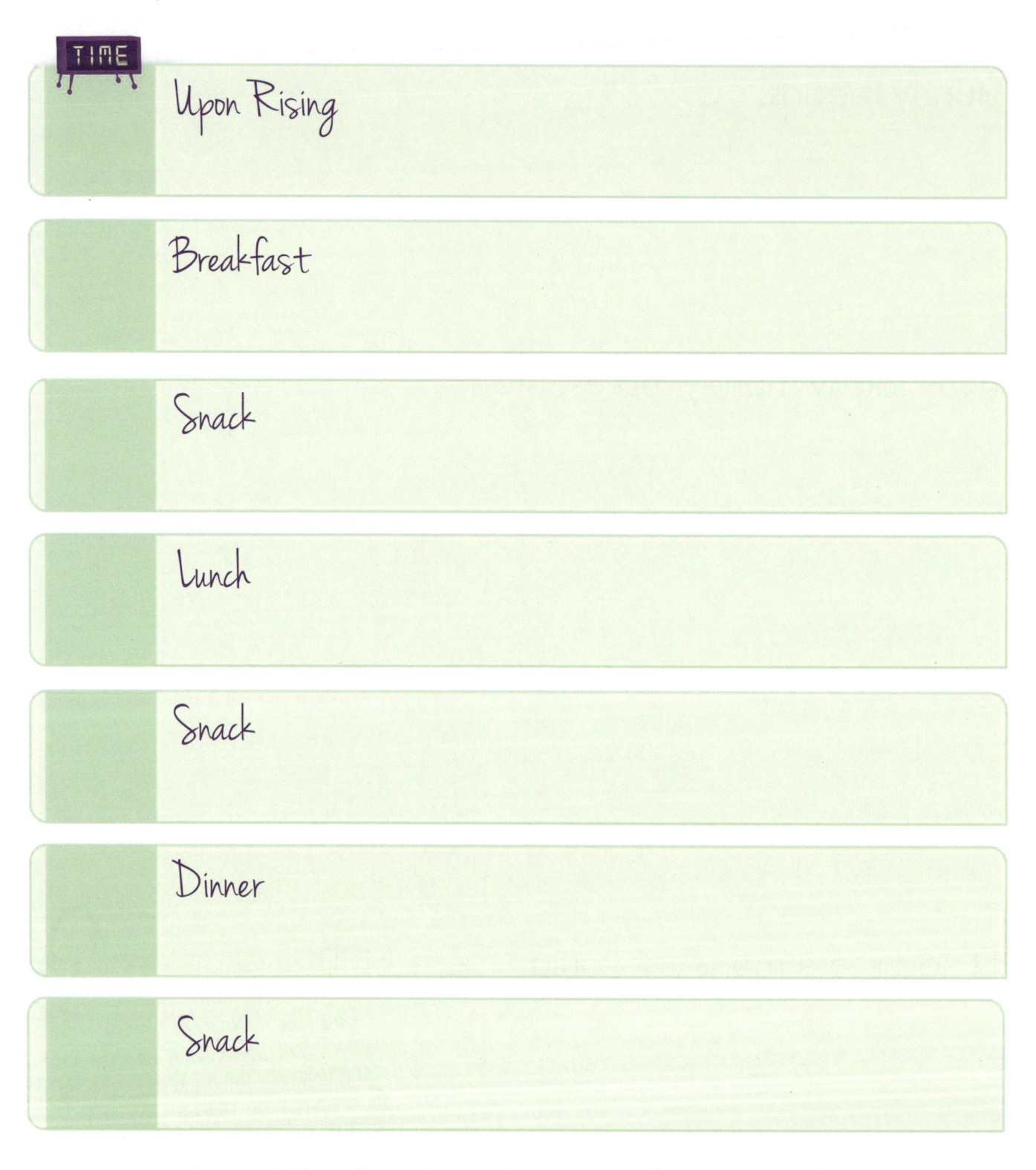

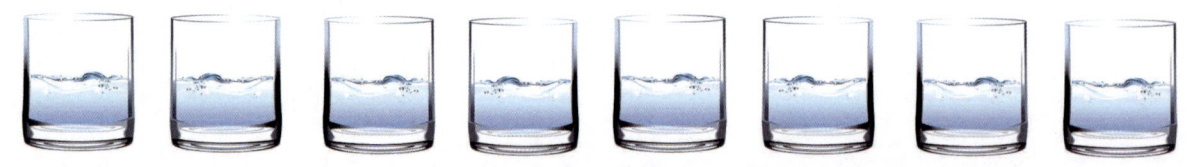

Week 3 — **Day 7**

TIME

Upon Rising

Breakfast

Snack

Lunch

Snack

Dinner

Snack

Place a check on the water cups to keep track of every 8oz you drink

Congrats!

You have made it to the end of the 3rd week. Time to check in with yourself.

1 How many days this week did you fill in your journal? Write the number, not the excuses.

Fill in the number of days be honest!

2 Biggest obstacles this week: List strategies for overcoming them.

....
....
....
....
....
....

3 What are your goals for the future?

....
....
....
....
....
....

We all know exercise is good for us - but why?

Exercise is any movement that gets your heart pumping, blood flowing and muscles engaged - and it should be fun. That's why PLAYING sports is more fun than WORKING out. Perhaps that's why most people think exercise is mundane, boring, or difficult. The problem is, if you hate doing something, you just don't do it - and then sadly, you see your middle growing, arms sagging and you're short of breath just climbing a flight of stairs. If you want to feel better, have more energy and perhaps even live longer - my suggestion is to fall in love with some form of daily exercise.

1. Exercise helps you manage your weight

Exercise causes your body to burn stored fat and burn calories. The more intense the activity, the more calories you burn and the easier it is to keep your weight under control. Try parking your car further away in a parking lot. Take a dance class or go roller skating. Maybe play tennis or swim - but if you want to lose it, move it!

2. Exercise boosts your energy level

Too often I hear, "I'm too tired to workout." My answer is, "if you want more energy, move!" As famed physicist Sir Isaac Newton stated, "an object in motion, tends to stay in motion;" same applies to you and your physical state. When you move, you help your body deliver oxygen and nutrients to your tissues; it also spikes various levels of brain chemicals that get you feeling energetic.

3. Exercise improves your mood

Physical activity stimulates various brain chemicals that may leave you feeling happier and more relaxed than before you worked out. You'll also look and feel better when you exercise regularly, which can boost your confidence and improve your self-esteem.

4. Exercise promotes better sleep

After a good night's sleep you feel better, your thoughts are clearer and you tend to have more energy throughout the day. Physical activity is sometimes the key to better sleep, may help you fall asleep faster and deepen your sleep. Just don't exercise too close to bedtime, as you may get too energized to nod off!

Try Something NEW

SpinGym is a compact and portable upper body fitness product (that I designed) to tone, strengthen, and sculpt. Unlike traditional training with dumbbells and weight machines, which isolate and target only one set of muscles at a time, SpinGym utilizes Gyrotronic Resistance Training (GRT) to simultaneously activate major, stabilizing and core muscles - all at the same time. With up to 20 lbs of resistance per pull, you feel the SpinGyms effect instantly and you only need 5-10 minutes a day to see a noticeable improvement. www.SpinGym.com

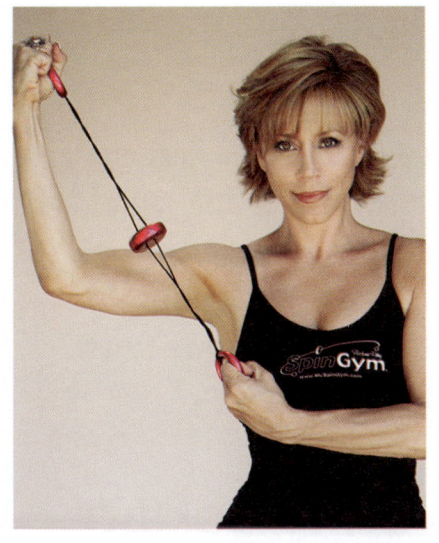

Forbes Riley, Creator of SpinGym

Rebounding is aerobic exercising on a mini trampoline. Unlike jogging on hard surfaces, which puts stress on certain joints such as ankles and knees, exercising on a rebounder is much lower impact. Trampolining uses gravity, acceleration and deceleration, forcing your body to cope with the conditions presented. Best of all, it is fun!

Pilates was developed in the early 1900's by fitness pioneer Joseph Pilates in Germany. Originally designed to help dancers rehabilitate their bodies, pilates is currently practiced by over 15 million people worldwide. The Pilates method can be practiced on a reformer (as pictured) or on the floor. It seeks to increase the flexibility and control of the body while emphasizing the concepts of core strength and stabilization.

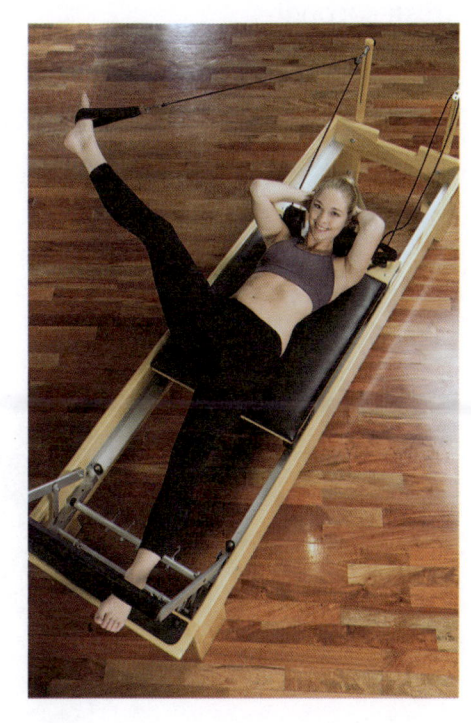

Fun & Healthy e.a.t. Recipe #3

Thai Twist Fruit Salad

> Healthy snacking in moderation with nutrient rich food is a part of a healthy diet. Some choices include almonds, olives, hummus, guacamole, and edamame. Fruit is also a great choice, but sometimes can be boring. This exotic combination of fruits is packed with nutrition, tastes delicious and will make you think you are eating dessert. Plan ahead - make this Thai Twist Fruit Salad and put it in the refrigerator for several hours before serving. Perfect for snacking and ideal adding zest to any party.

For a fresh refreshing exotic twist on snacking...

Ingredients

- Half a honeydew melon
- Half a pineapple
- A quarter of a watermelon
- 1 star fruit
- 2 oz of coconut flakes or 4oz fresh coconut
- 4 passion fruit
- Juice of 2 limes

Directions

1. Peel and slice the pineapple into bite size chunks. Scoop out the seeds of the honeydew and slice into bite size chunks. Cut the watermelon into chunks, discarding any seeds. Cut the star fruit into four and slice thin.

2. In a large bowl toss together the pineapple, honeydew melon, watermelon, star fruit and coconut. Halve the passion fruits and scoop out the pulp into a separate bowl. Mix in the lime juice and toss together. Cover and chill for 4 hours before serving. This fruit salad is rich in vitamin C, potassium and fiber. Also rich in lycopene and antioxidants. Refreshing and exotic with a hint of lime - you'll feel like you're on an exotic vacation.

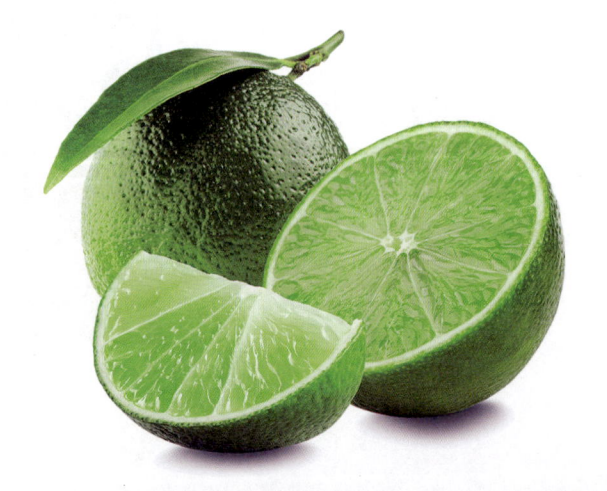

Here's to Your Health - Word Jumble

"Be the change you want to see" In this Word Jumble unscramble the letters to reveal words that will continue to remind you about healthy food and lifestyle choices - it's a quick break from your day, but helps keep you focused on your goal. Enjoy!

eabevltgse _____	linrjaou _____
fnsiste _____	uscssec _____
ruwkoost _____	niripnioastn _____
ragaspusa _____	hylpsica _____
omlesn _____	gnorst _____
cckhien _____	lrecosetlho _____
keast _____	tmaiinvs _____
floiueraclw _____	igracon _____
tceleut _____	utlrnaa _____
iwsrfdhso _____	elaeirthh _____
tttiaeud _____	tarwe _____

One should live to eat, not eat to live.

- Moliere

Congratulations

You're 1/2 way through the e.a.t. transformational journal program 3 weeks down, 3 more to go!

First we make our habits, then our habits make us.

- Charles C. Noble

Week 4

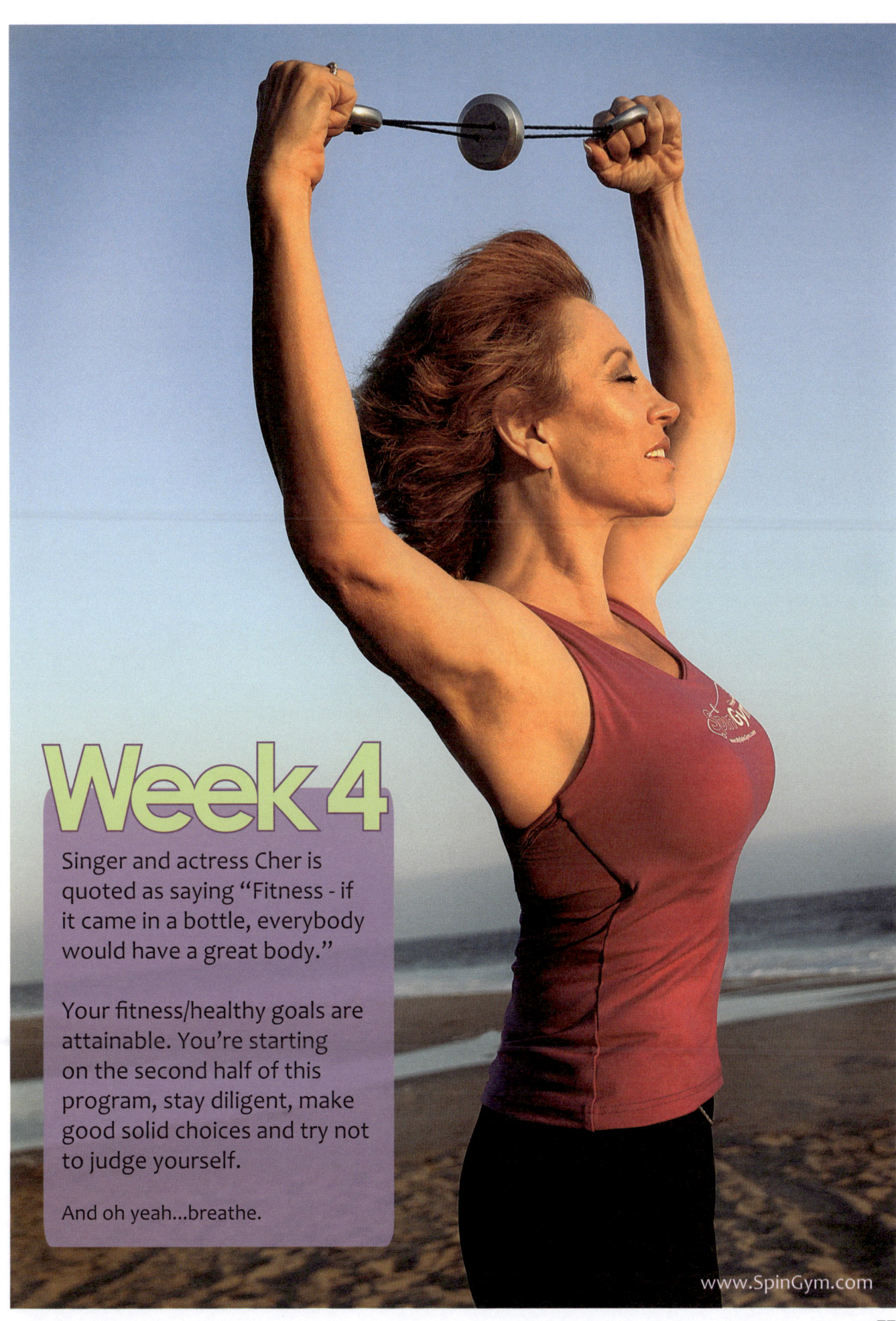

Singer and actress Cher is quoted as saying "Fitness - if it came in a bottle, everybody would have a great body."

Your fitness/healthy goals are attainable. You're starting on the second half of this program, stay diligent, make good solid choices and try not to judge yourself.

And oh yeah...breathe.

www.SpinGym.com

What I Eat

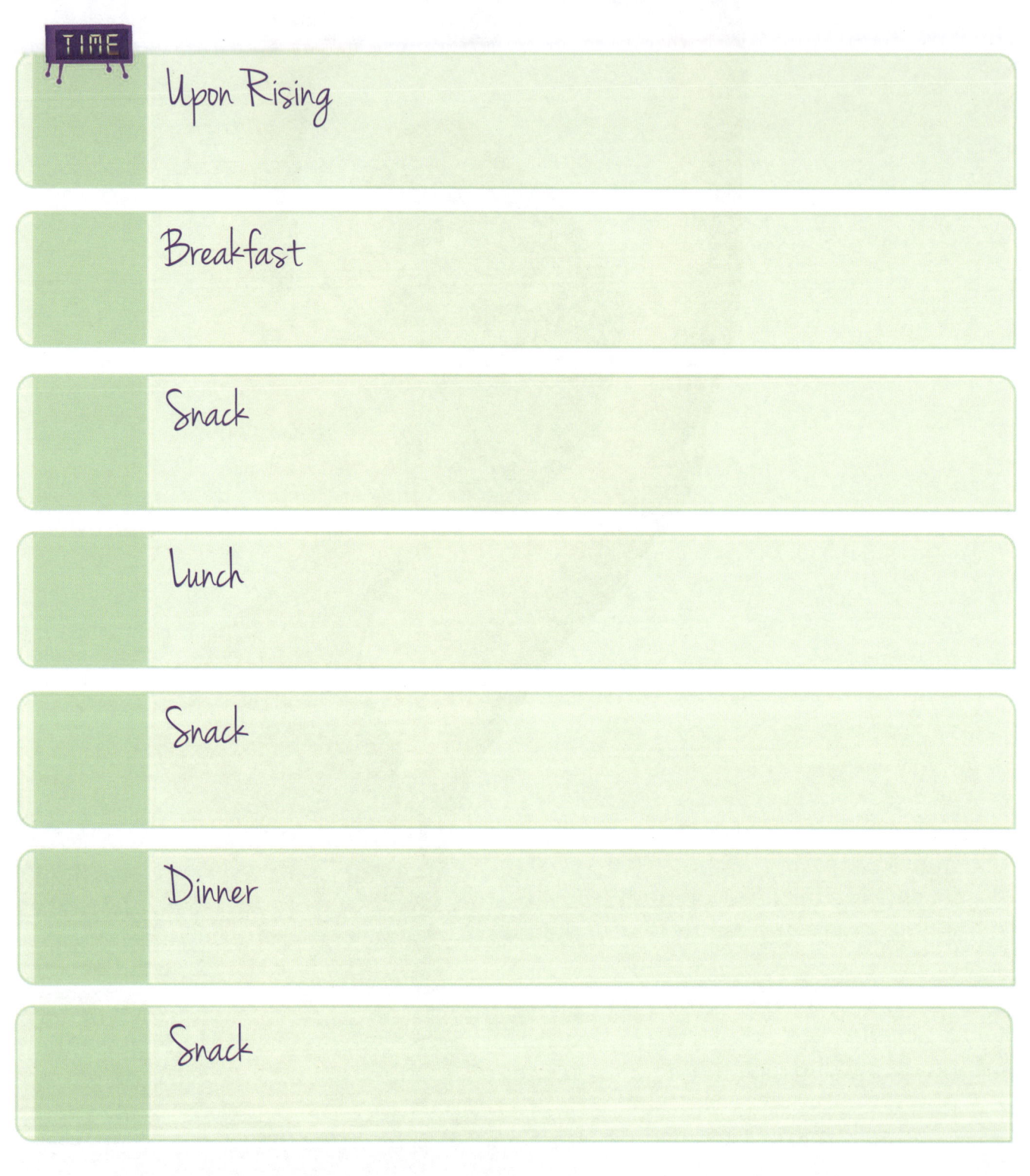

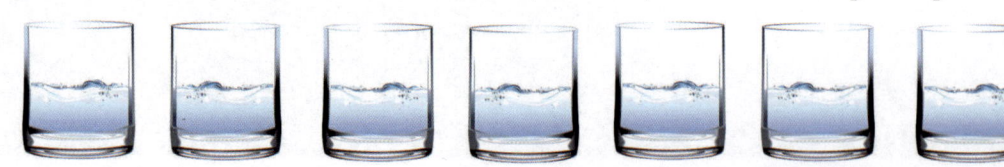

Week 4 — **Day 1**

TIME

Upon Rising

Breakfast

Snack

Lunch

Snack

Dinner

Snack

Place a check on the water cups to keep track of every 8oz you drink

Don't Give Up

Sometimes the hardest part of any journey is the home stretch, but it can also be the most rewarding. Here we are, halfway through the program - don't give up now!

What are 3 of your best achievements so far?

1

2

3

> **Tip**
>
> Try a vegetable you've never had before. Experiment with eggplant, kale, bean sprouts, bok choy, or fennel. Try adding these unique and nutritious foods to a salad or stir fry.
>
> Be adventurous.

Week 4 # What I Eat **Day 2**

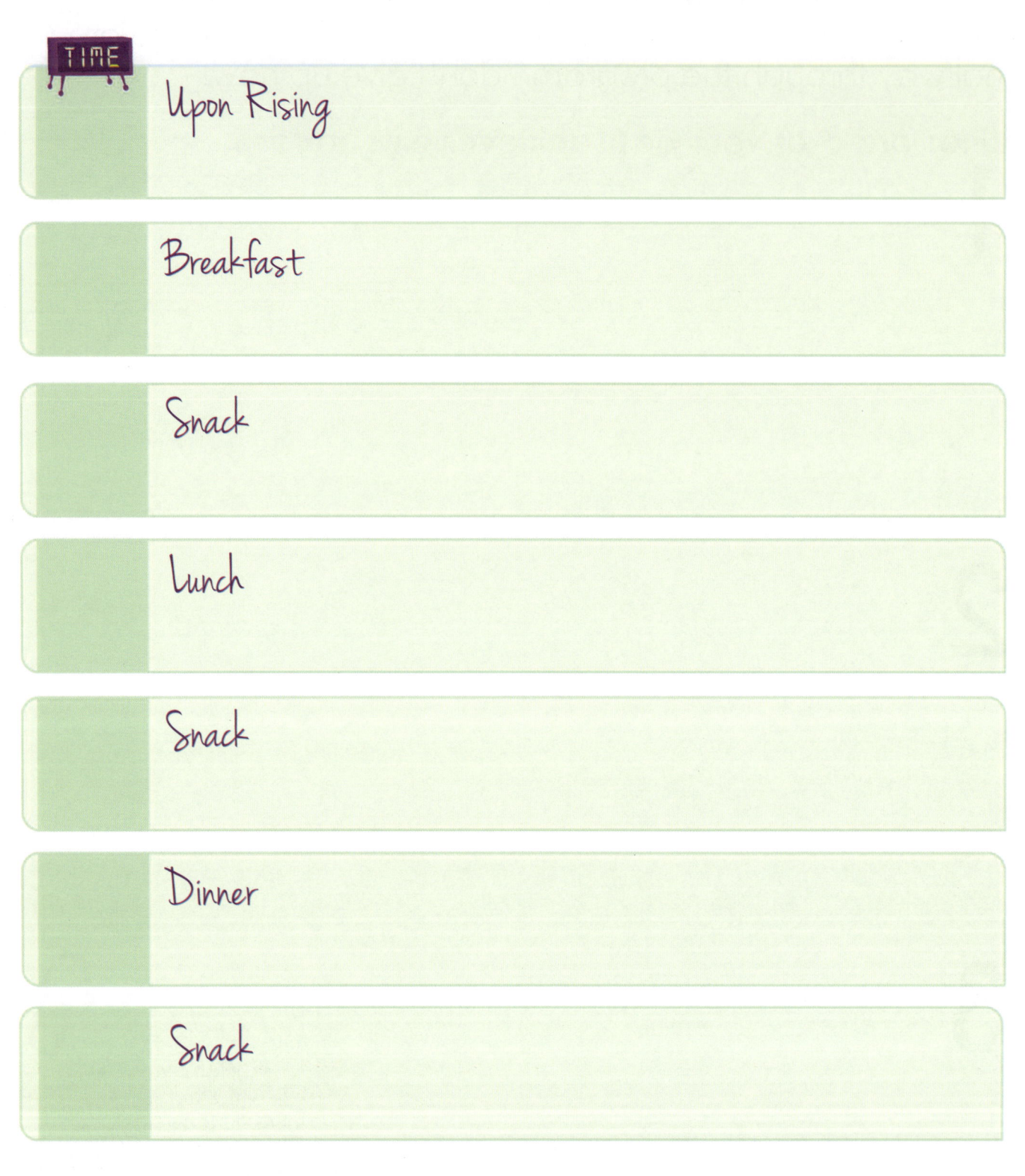

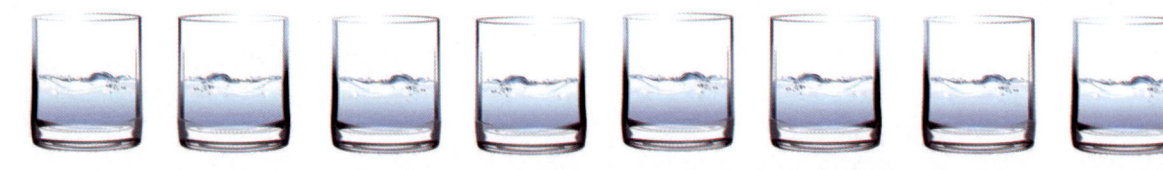

TIME

Upon Rising

Breakfast

Snack

Lunch

Snack

Dinner

Snack

Place a check on the water cups to keep track of every 8oz you drink

80

Focus (Foh-kuhs) noun

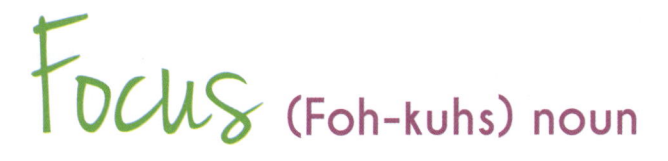

1. A central point of attraction, attention or activity
2. To concentrate or to bring into

What are you choosing to focus on today?

What are you striving to become & why?

> **TIP**
>
> Water, water everywhere. Try drinking water as your only beverage for the entire day. You will be surprised how good you will feel and how much brighter your skin will look.

What I Eat

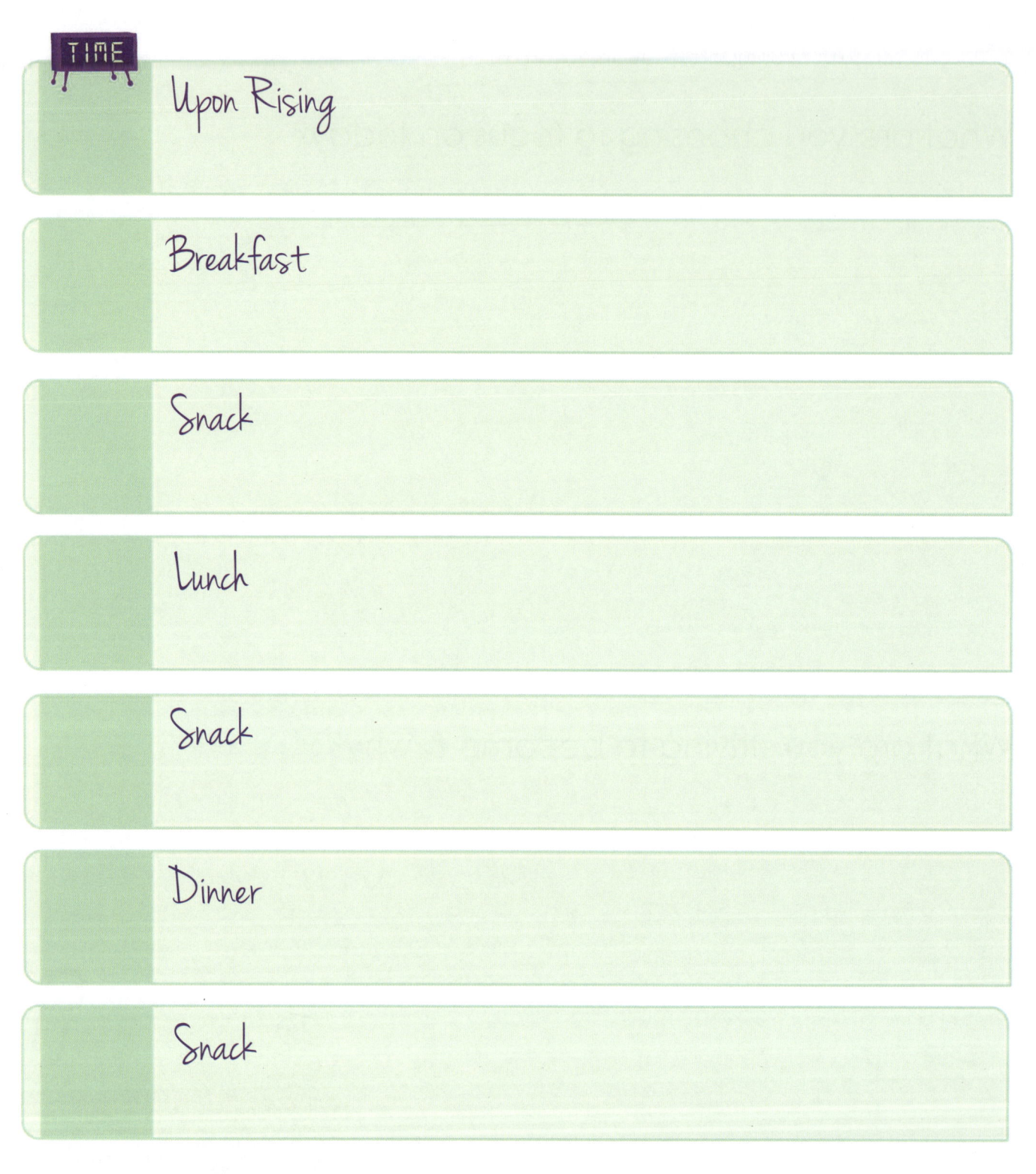

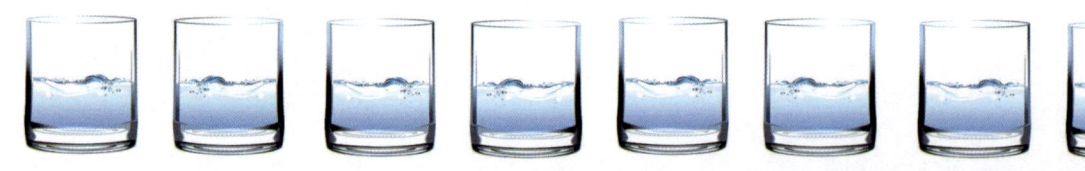

Week 4 — **Day 3**

TIME

- Upon Rising
- Breakfast
- Snack
- Lunch
- Snack
- Dinner
- Snack

Place a check on the water cups to keep track of every 8oz you drink

List your **5 favorite movies**. Any common themes? Romance, thrillers, adventures?

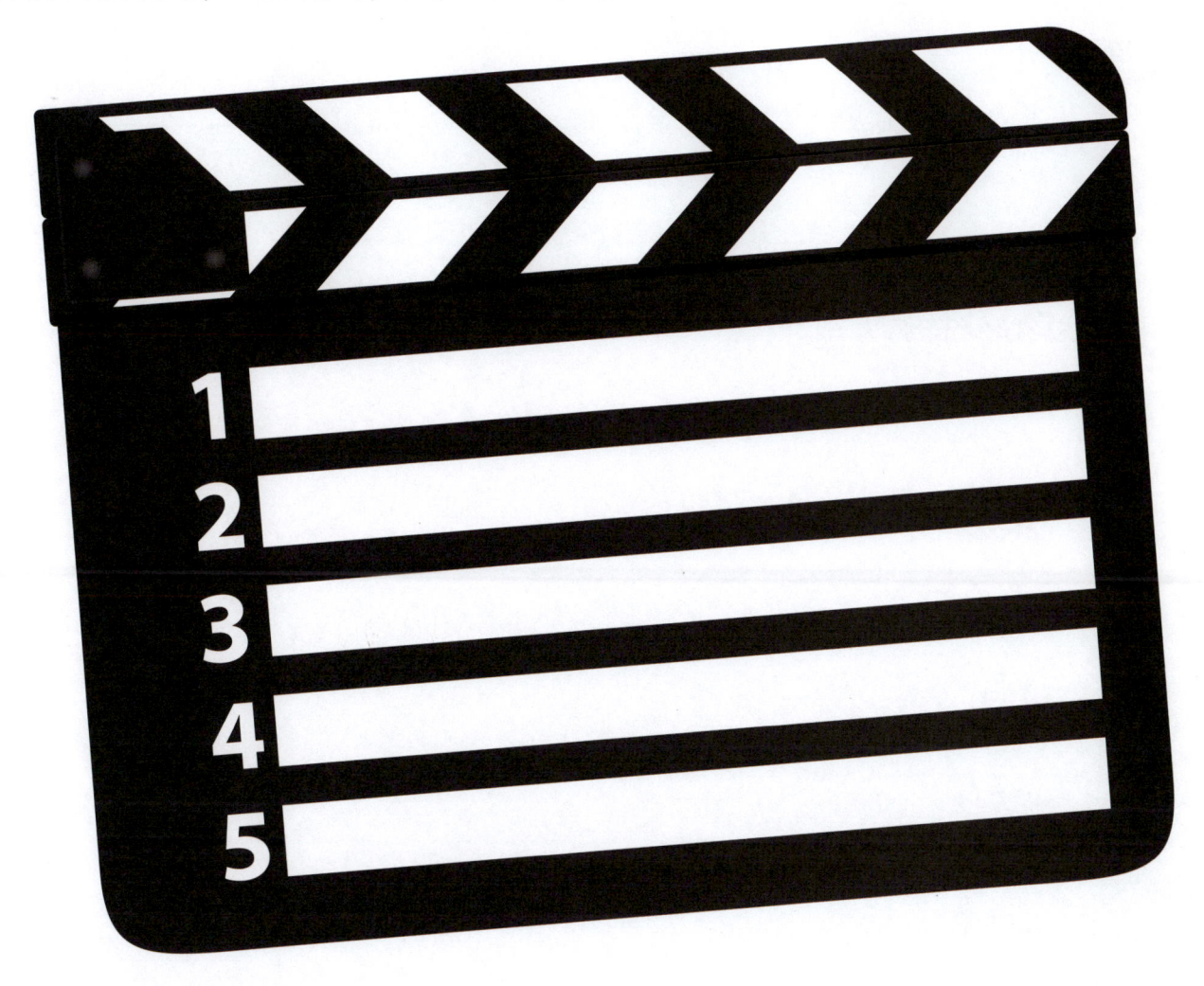

1.
2.
3.
4.
5.

Describe yourself as a character in one of your favorite films.

Create your life to be Oscar worthy!

Week 4 # What I Eat **Day 4**

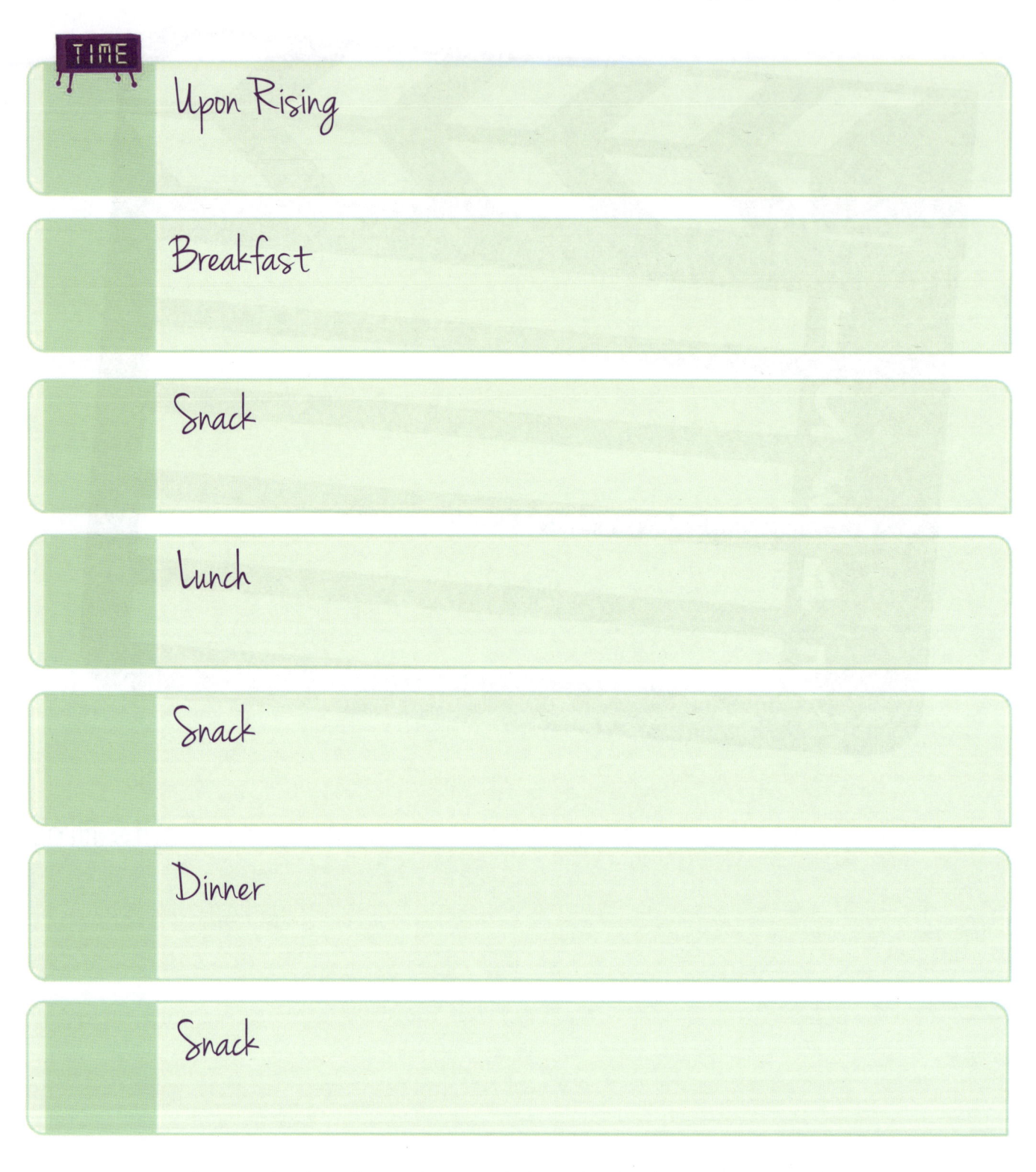

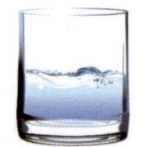

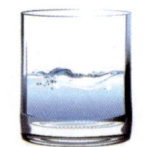

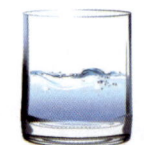

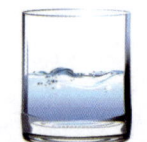

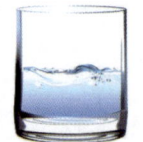

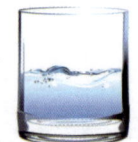

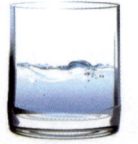

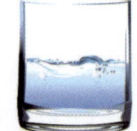

TIME

Upon Rising

Breakfast

Snack

Lunch

Snack

Dinner

Snack

Place a check on the water cups to keep track of every 8oz you drink

Taboos.
Things we are not allowed to do, but secretly wish we could. Write 3 things that are taboo for you

For example: skinny dipping, buying $300 shoes, visiting your hometown and not telling your relatives.

1 ......
2 ......
3 ......

Imagine yourself doing one of them and write about how that experience may feel.

....
....
....
....
....
....
....
....

> **Tip**
> Chew.
>
> Chewing your food is directly connected with the movement of food through your digestive tract. Chewing thoroughly aids in the proper transport of nutrients...
> so chew on that!

What I Eat

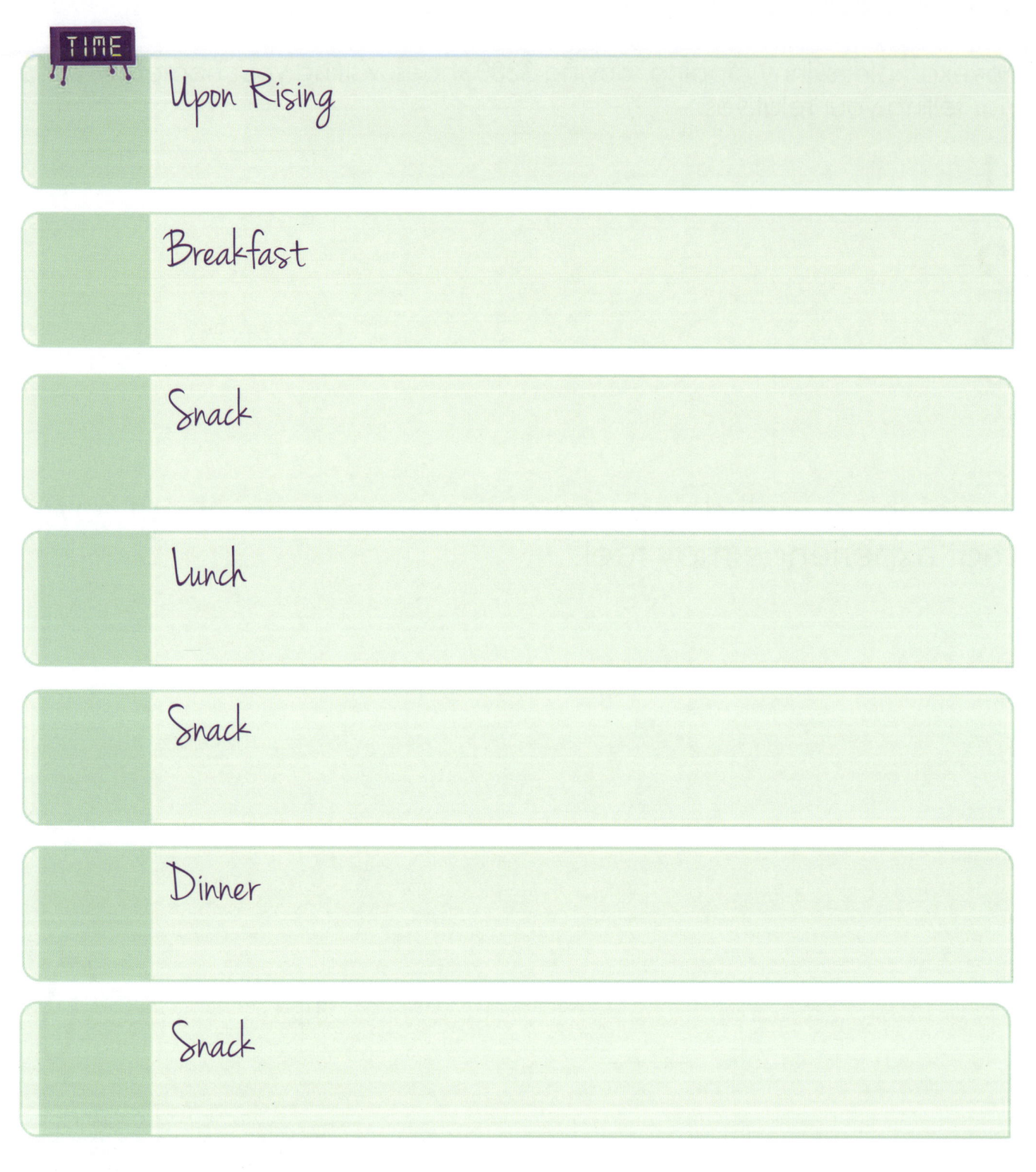

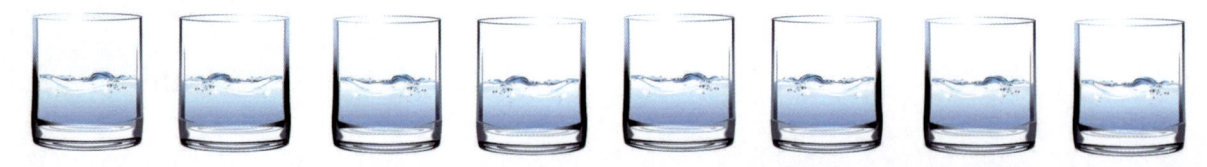

Week 4 — **Day 5**

TIME

- Upon Rising
- Breakfast
- Snack
- Lunch
- Snack
- Dinner
- Snack

Place a check on the water cups to keep track of every 8oz you drink

List **5 things** that you tend to beat yourself up about.

1. ....
2. ....
3. ....
4. ....
5. ....

How can you change one of them?

....
....
....
....
....
....
....

Be honest, will you change?

☐ Yes   ☐ No

When? ___ / ___ / ___ (date)

What I Eat

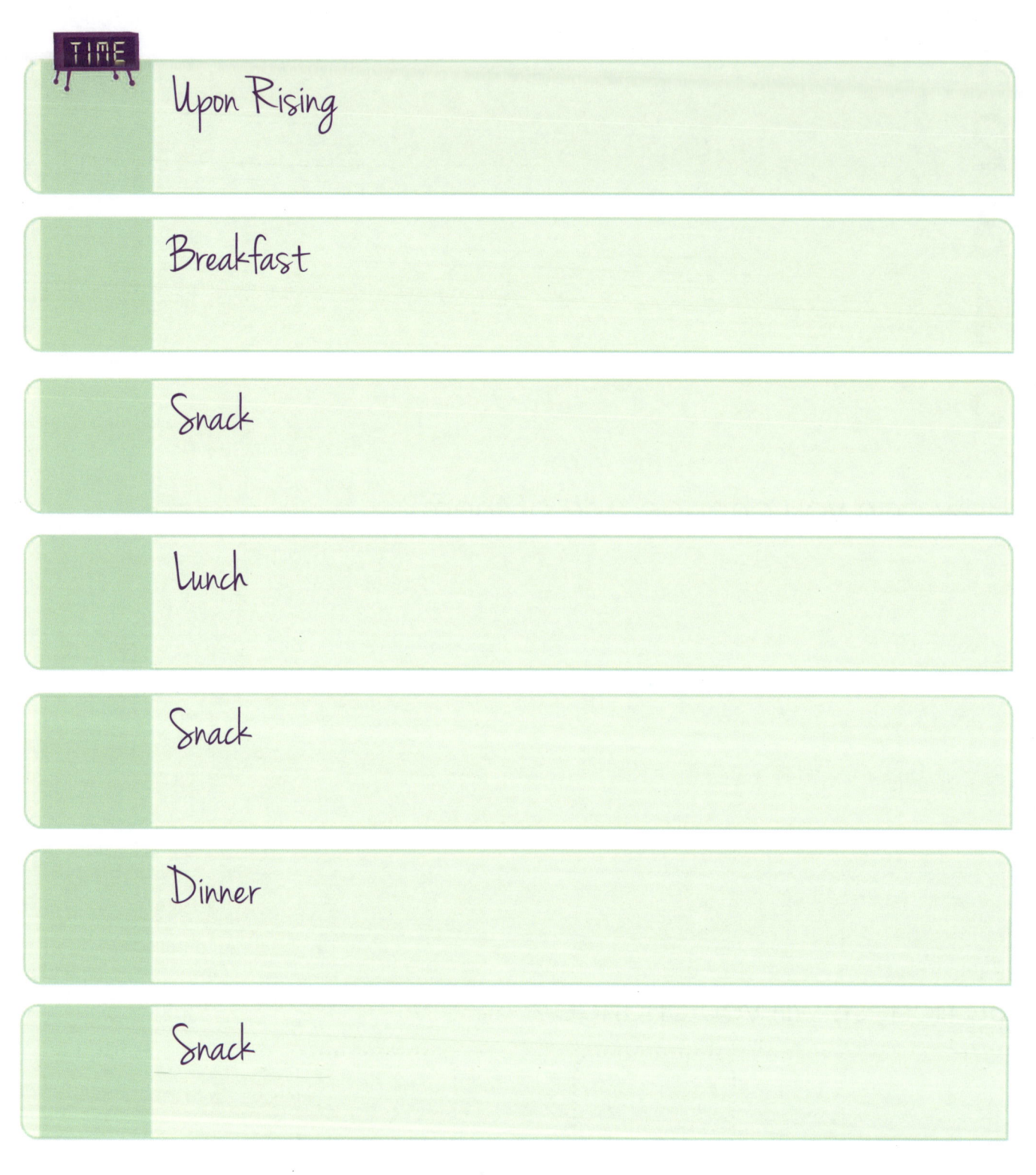

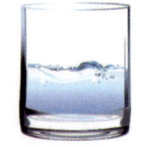

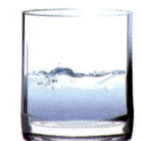

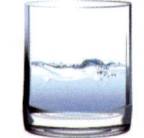

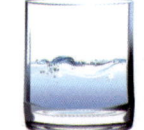

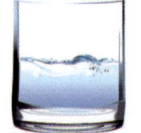

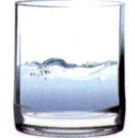

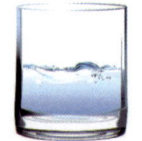

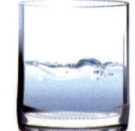

Week 4 — Day 6

TIME

Upon Rising

Breakfast

Snack

Lunch

Snack

Dinner

Snack

Place a check on the water cups to keep track of every 8oz you drink

Change occupations

Imagine for a moment that you did something else for a living, even if you love what you do. Describe this new occupation and why you chose it.

> **Tip**
>
> Enzymes – sprouted seeds, raw vegetables, raw fruits and soaked nuts are loaded with live enzymes – one of the keys to vibrant health. Once our food is cooked, the enzymes are destroyed. Try eating more raw and sprouted foods.

What I Eat

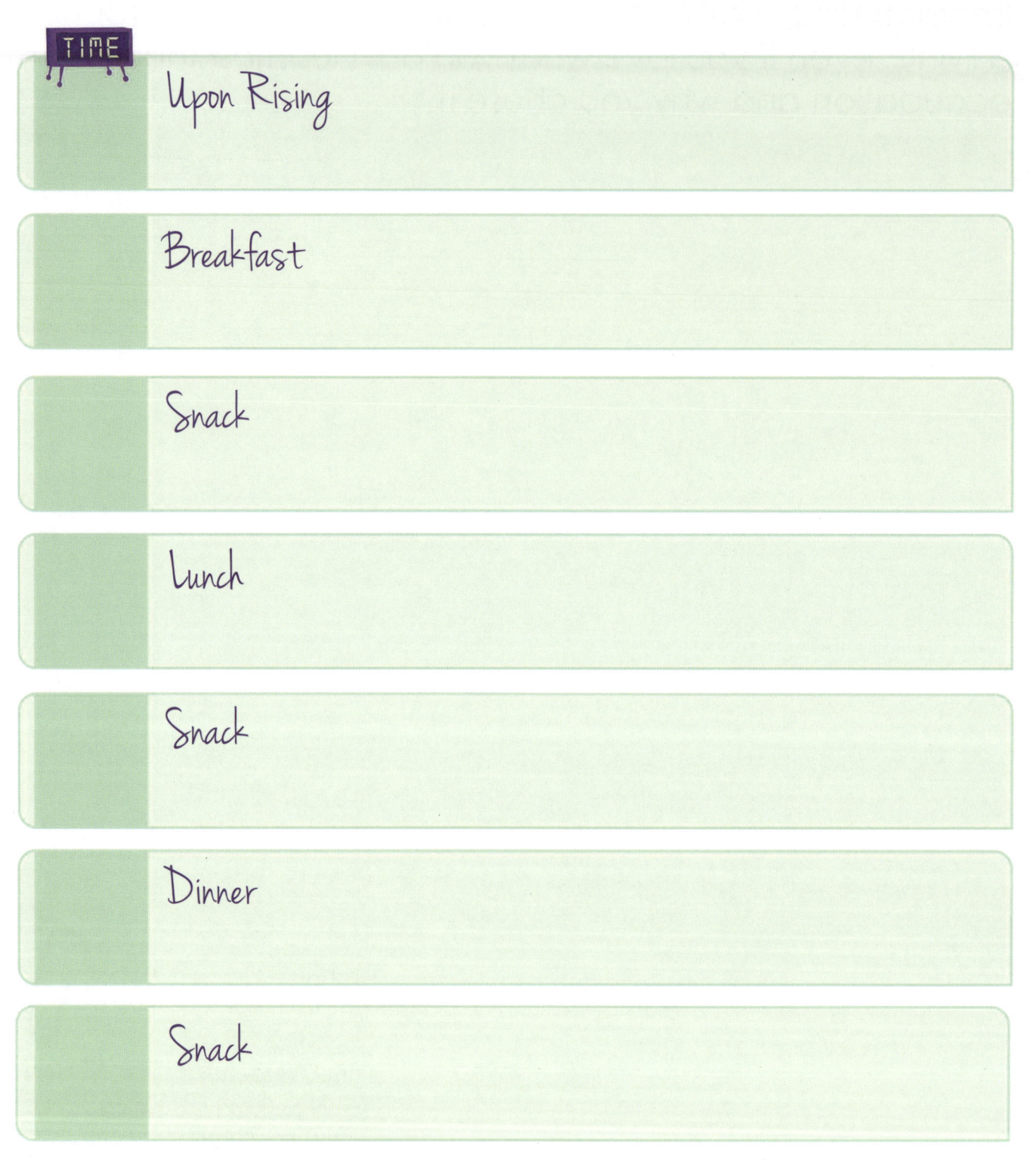

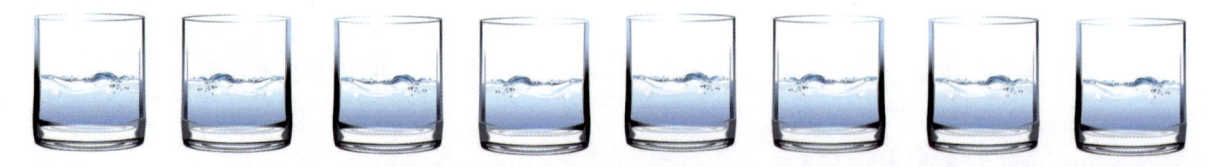

Week 4 — Day 7

TIME

Upon Rising

Breakfast

Snack

Lunch

Snack

Dinner

Snack

Place a check on the water cups to keep track of every 8oz you drink

Congrats!

You have made it to the end of the 4th week. Time to check in with yourself.

1 How many days this week did you fill in your journal? Write the number, not the excuses.

> Fill in the number of days
> *be honest!*

2 Biggest obstacles this week:
List strategies for overcoming them.

....
....
....
....
....
....

3 What are your goals for the future?

....
....
....
....
....
....

Fun & Healthy e.a.t. Recipe # 4

Vegetable Soup

If you are having trouble getting all your veggies into your diet daily - stealth 'em. Sneak vegetables into a soup, it's an easy and nutritious way to get in your daily requirement of 5 or 6 of them. Soup, whether clear or thick, is a great staple food and should be incorporated on a regular basis into a healthy diet. There is such a variety from the traditional chicken soup, to the veggie rich minestrone, pea soup, to meat and rice barley. This recipe incorporates legumes - a rich source of protein, complex carbohydrates and fiber. They provide a slow burning fuel and keep you feeling full.

Soups On!

Ingredients

- 1 1/2 cups of mixed dried beans (black beans, navy beans and kidney beans
- 1/2 cup of lentils
- 1/2 cup of split peas
- 1/3 cup of barley
- 2 cooking onions (chopped)
- 3 large carrots (peeled and chopped)
- 4 celery stalks
- 10 cups low-sodium chicken broth
- 3 cups of stewed plum tomatoes
- 1/4 tsp dried and crumbled thyme leaves
- 1 bay leaf
- 1/2 tsp coarsely ground pepper
- 2 gloves of garlic, roasted
- 1/2 cup fresh chopped parsley
- 2 cups Water

Directions

1. Put dried beans in a large saucepan and cover with water. Bring to a rolling boil over high heat, uncovered. Remove from heat and cover. Let sit for one hour.

2. Drain, Rinse barley, lentils and split peas. Drain. In large saute pan, add onions, celery and carrots. Add broth, tomatoes (and their juice), seasonings, beans, lentils, split peas and barley.

3. Boil. Cover and reduce heat to low. Cook, stirring occasionally until beans and vegetables are tender - approx. 2 hours. Add roasted garlic.

4. Simmer for another 5 minutes. Add chopped parsley and serve.

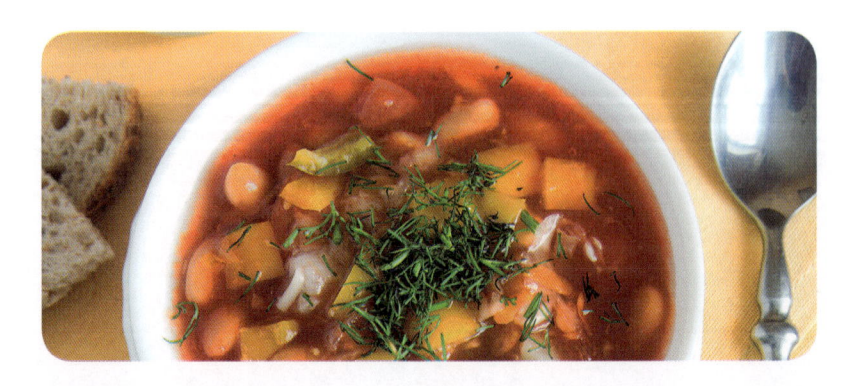

Forbes Fit & Fun

Fill in the missing letters to reveal your new lifestyle.

ARTIC(H)OKES

B(E)ETS

M(A)NGOES

P(L)UMS

LET(T)UCE

C(H)ERRIES

PAPA(Y)AS

(C)ABBAGE

ZUCC(H)INI

LEM(O)NS

K(I)WI

BROC(C)OLI

WATERM(E)LON

(S)QUASH

Let's make 'em...

_ _ _ _ _ _ _   _ _ _ _ _ _ _ _

93

Notes

> If man made it, don't eat it.
>
> - Jack LaLanne

Week 5

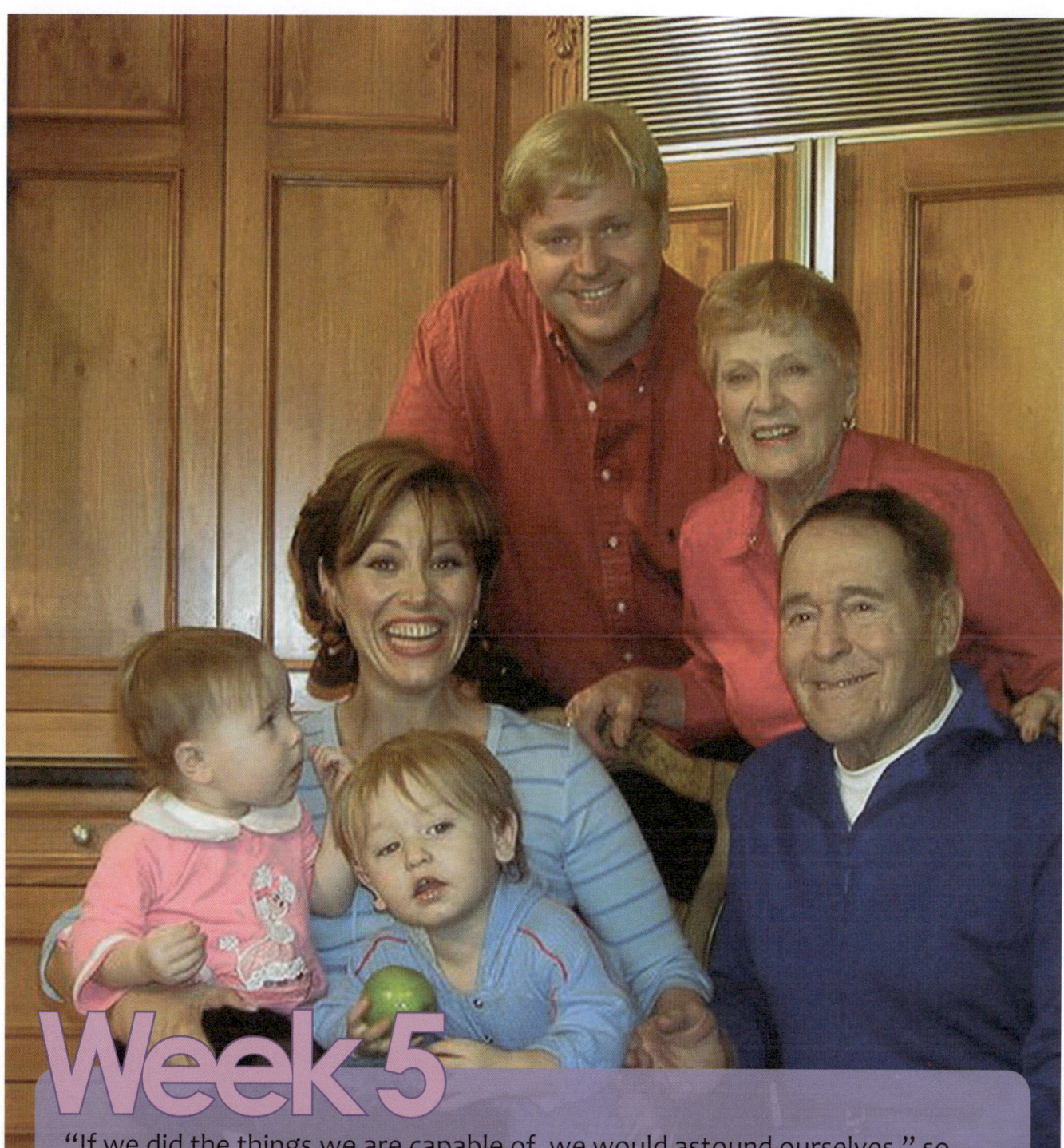

"If we did the things we are capable of, we would astound ourselves," so said Thomas Edison. A man who also said, "I have not failed. I have just found 10,000 ways that won't work." As you approach the finish line of this journey, don't let the perfect ruin the good.

Perhaps you missed a day or two of journal writing, or did not complete one of the exercises. Don't judge or beat yourself up, simply take a breath and renew your commitment to yourself and to your goals.

Forbes, Tom & twins Ryker & Makenna (6 months) visiting with Elaine and Jack LaLanne

What I Eat

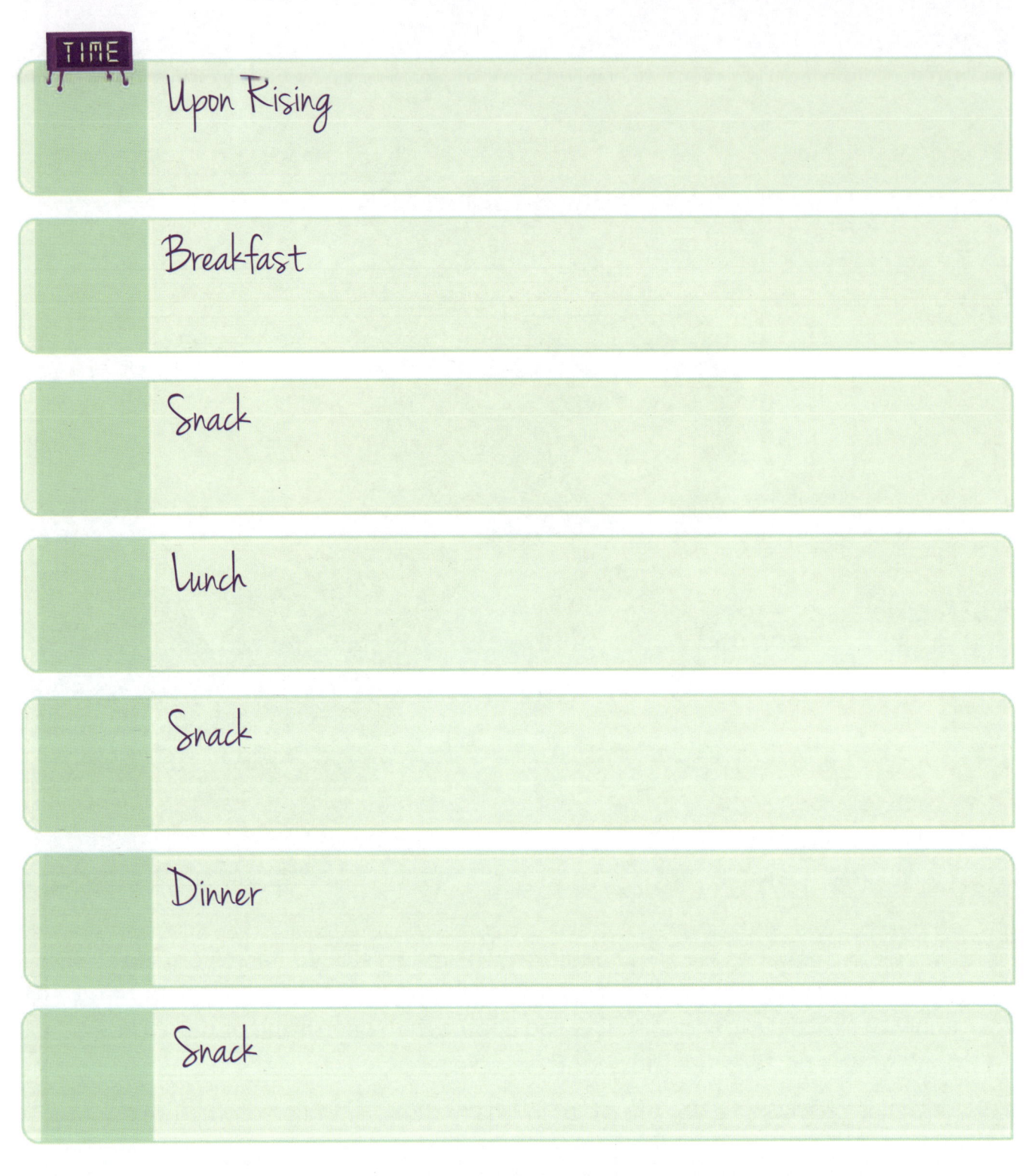

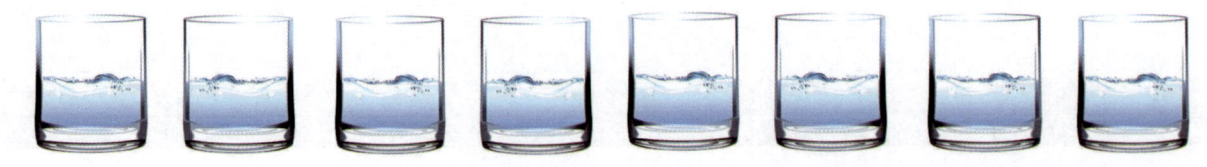

Week 5 — **Day 1**

TIME

- Upon Rising
- Breakfast
- Snack
- Lunch
- Snack
- Dinner
- Snack

Place a check on the water cups to keep track of every 8oz you drink

Dare to Risk.

Risk is defined as "doing something outside of the box." For this page, imagine stepping outside of your comfort zone. For example: speaking in public, volunteering at a nursing home, or eating dinner alone at a restaurant, quitting a job you hate, or leaving a destructive relationship.

Push your personal limits and describe a risk that you can imagine tackling. A risk that gets your heart pumping, palms sweating and is worth daring to do!

TIP

Laughter has been known to lessen tension, deepen breathing and exercises internal muscles. So rent a comedy video or watch your favorite sitcom.

Have a good laugh.

What I Eat

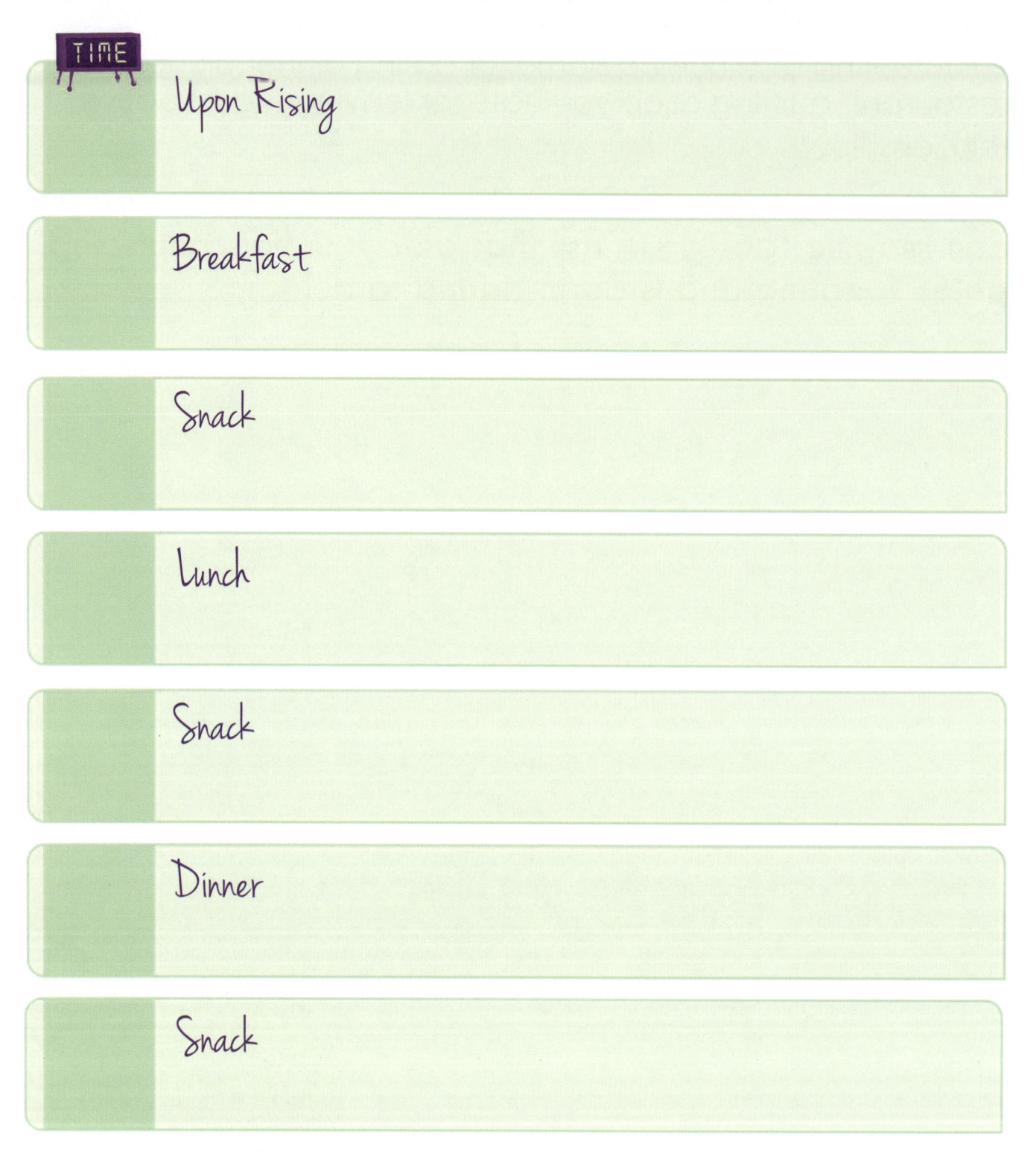

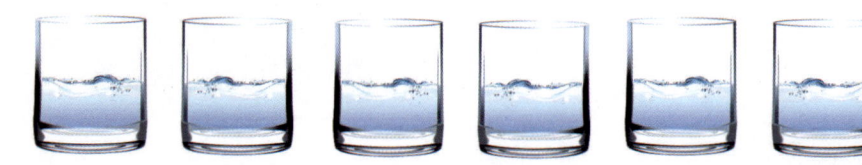

Week 5 — **Day 2**

TIME

- Upon Rising
- Breakfast
- Snack
- Lunch
- Snack
- Dinner
- Snack

Place a check on the water cups to keep track of every 8oz you drink

It's often said "no news is good news," but in today's day and age, we're on information overload. Describe a current event that is affecting you emotionally, good or bad. Go on... Write!

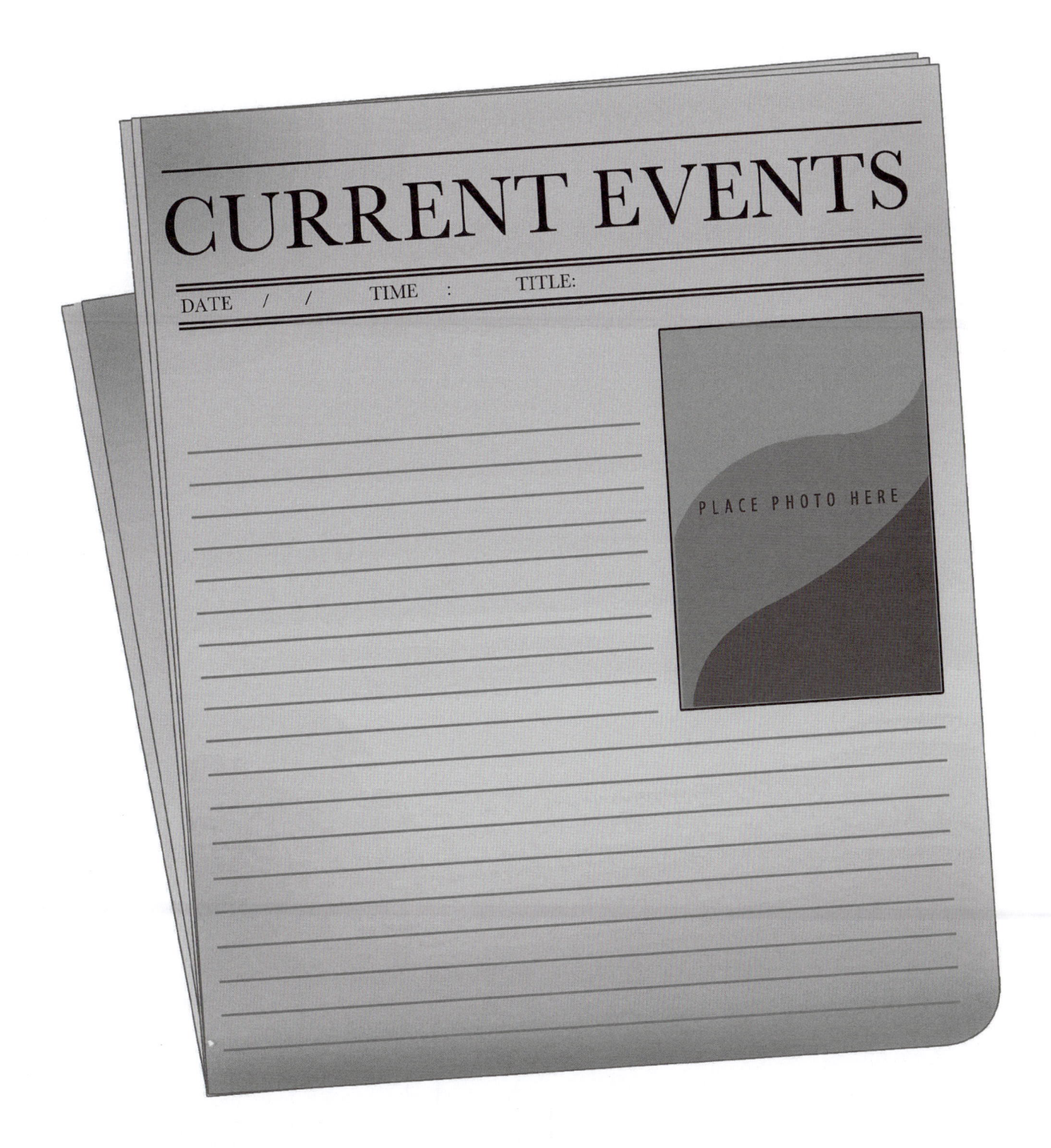

CURRENT EVENTS

DATE / / TIME : TITLE:

PLACE PHOTO HERE

What I Eat

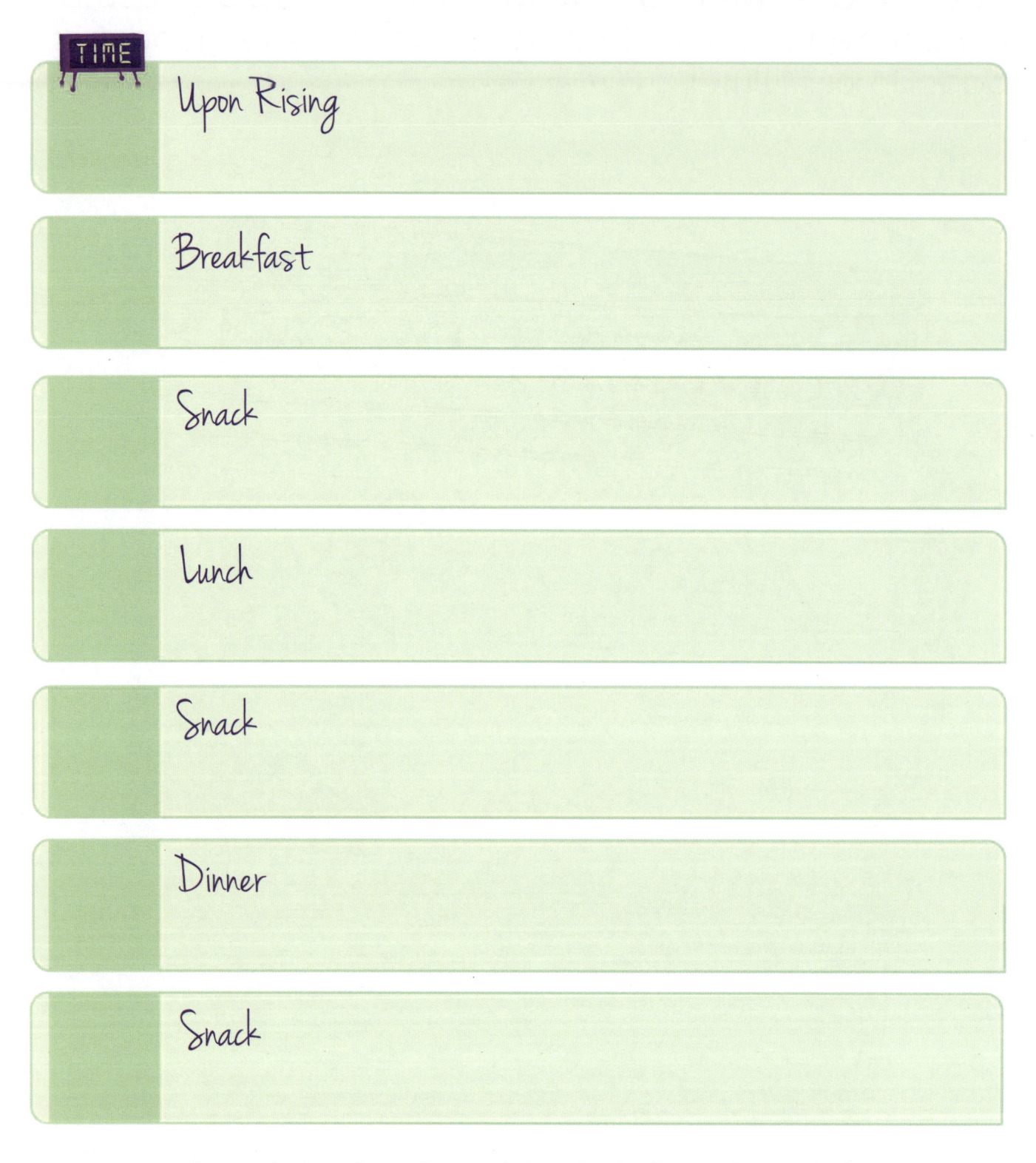

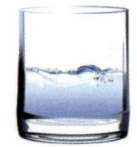

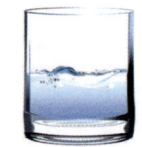

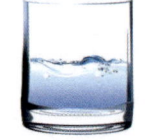

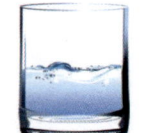

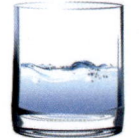

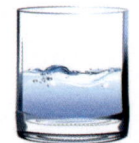

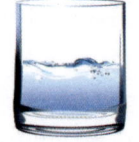

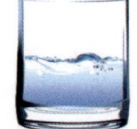

Week 5 **Day 3**

TIME

Upon Rising

Breakfast

Snack

Lunch

Snack

Dinner

Snack

Place a check on the water cups to keep track of every 8oz you drink

Interview your favorite movie star. Write down 3 questions and what their answers might be. Why are you such a fan?

1

2

3

Tip
Celebrate! Rather than celebrating with food- treat yourself with a massage, pedicure or manicure. Pampering yourself can make you feell extra special.

Week 5 — What I Eat — **Day 4**

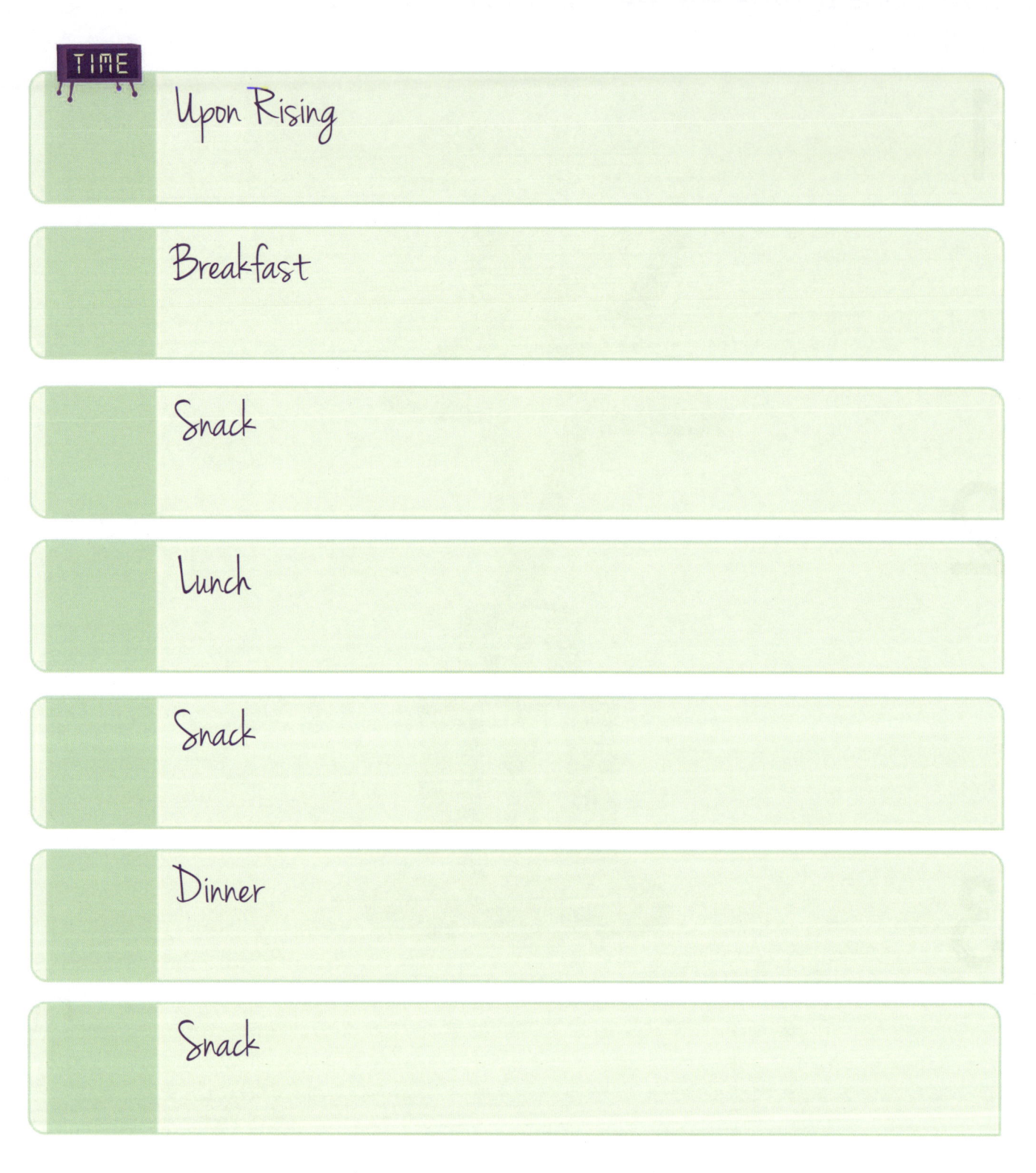

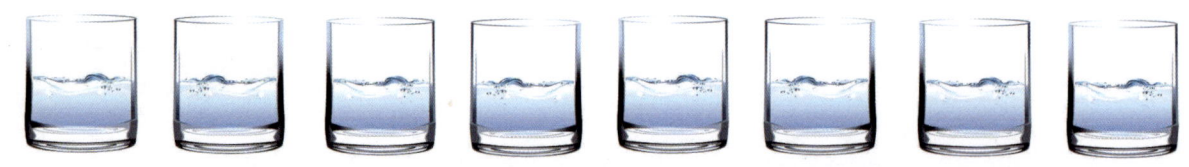

TIME

- Upon Rising
- Breakfast
- Snack
- Lunch
- Snack
- Dinner
- Snack

Place a check on the water cups to keep track of every 8oz you drink

Visualize (vizh-oo-uh-lahyz) verb

1. To recall or form mental images or ideas.
2. to make perceptible to the mind or imagination.

Imagination and thoughts are the tools of success. Close your eyes and visualize your ideal body. What does it look like? What is it wearing? What is it doing? Open your eyes and fill this page with your thoughts.

> **Tip**
>
> As a snack, try edamame. They are soy beans and an excellent source of protein; they are also packed with Vitamin C, calcium and iron. Commonly found in Japanese restaurants, they are available in most grocery stores. Healthy and low calorie, they make a great appetizer.

What I Eat

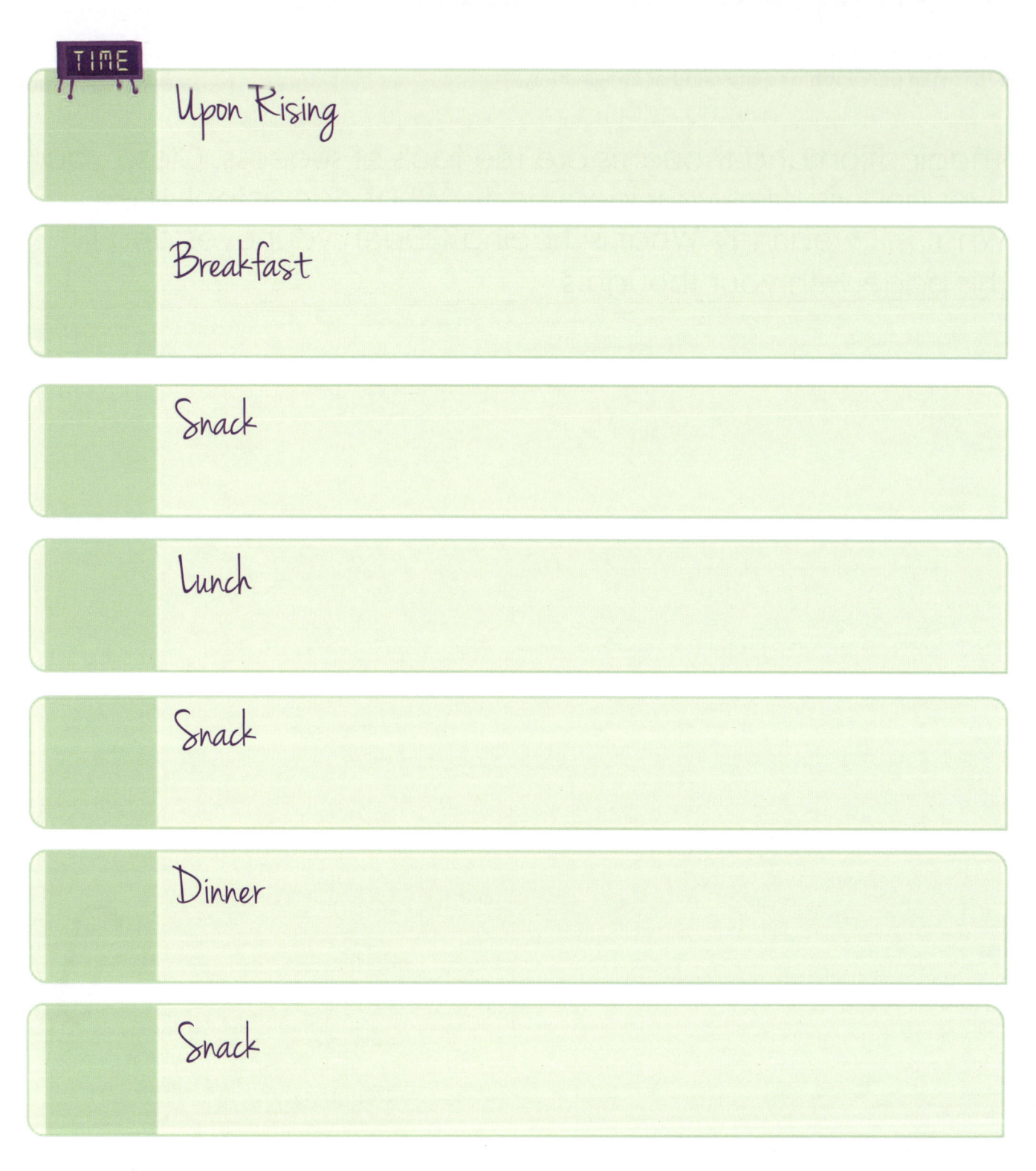

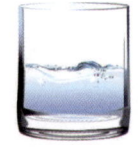

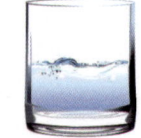

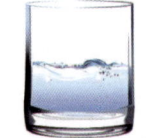

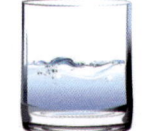

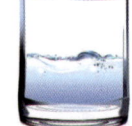

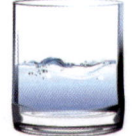

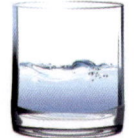

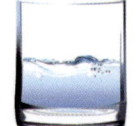

Week 5 — **Day 5**

TIME	
	Upon Rising
	Breakfast
	Snack
	Lunch
	Snack
	Dinner
	Snack

Place a check on the water cups to keep track of every 8oz you drink

A **Vision Board** is a simple yet powerful visualization tool that activates the universal Law of Attraction to begin manifesting your dreams into reality. A Vision Board is a visual representation or collage of the things you want to have, be or do in your life. Cut out several pictures from magazines that represent your dreams and place them on a poster board.

Use the space below to write several of the key ideas you will be looking for when creating your vision board...

What I Eat

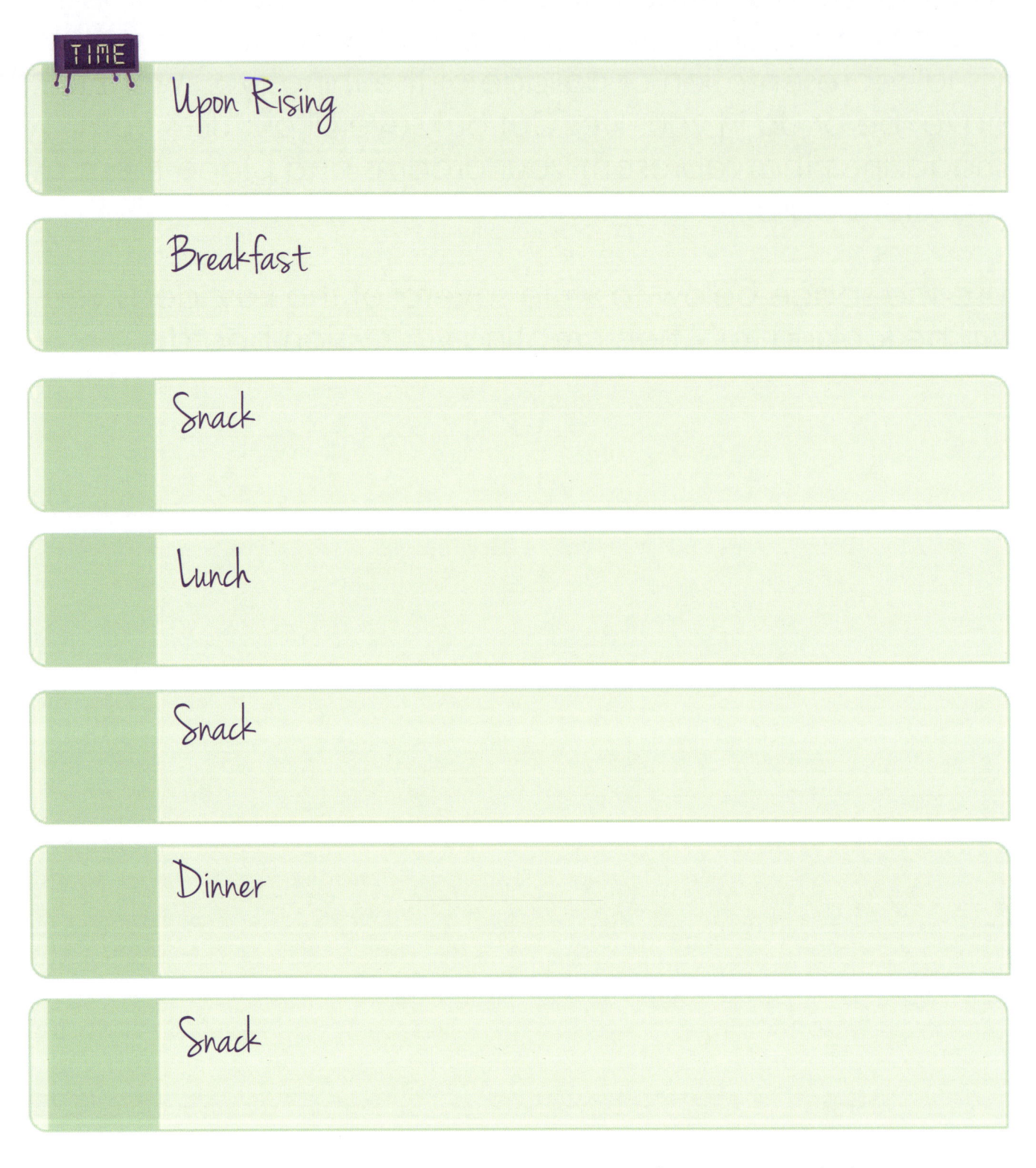

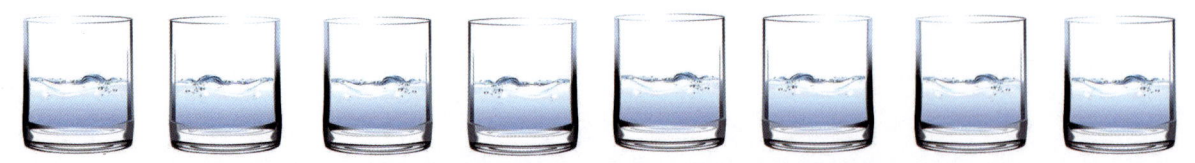

Week 5 — **Day 6**

TIME

- Upon Rising
- Breakfast
- Snack
- Lunch
- Snack
- Dinner
- Snack

Place a check on the water cups to keep track of every 8oz you drink

Create your own *Vision Board* on a giant piece of cardboard or corkboard. Clip photos to inspire and motivate you. Draw or write words that help you imagine what your life can be. This is a place to dream, be colorful, be creative.

> Below is a sample Vision Board. When creating your own, refer to your key ideas on page 107.

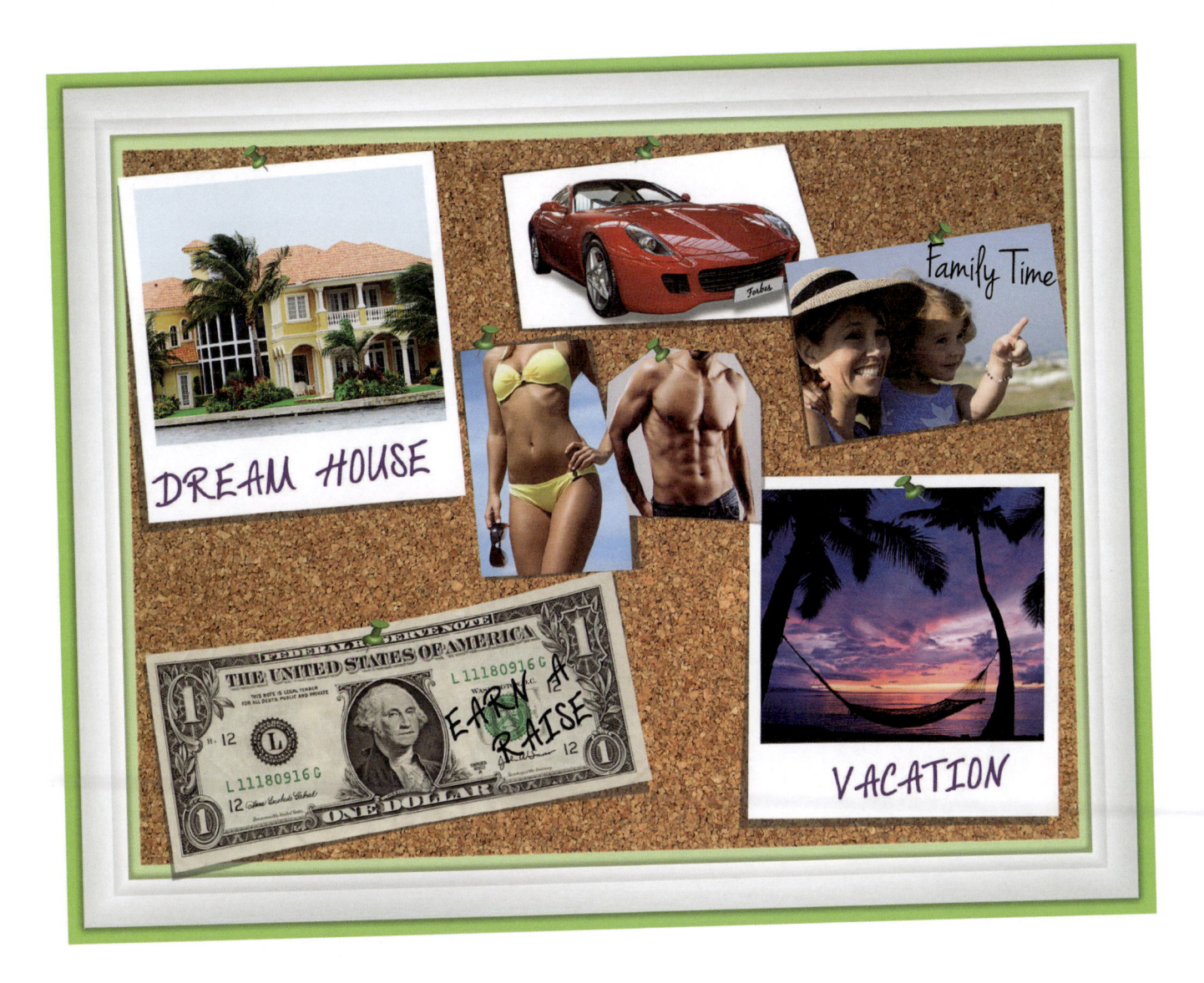

P.S. A Vision Board should be placed where you will see it daily!

Week 5 # What I Eat **Day 7**

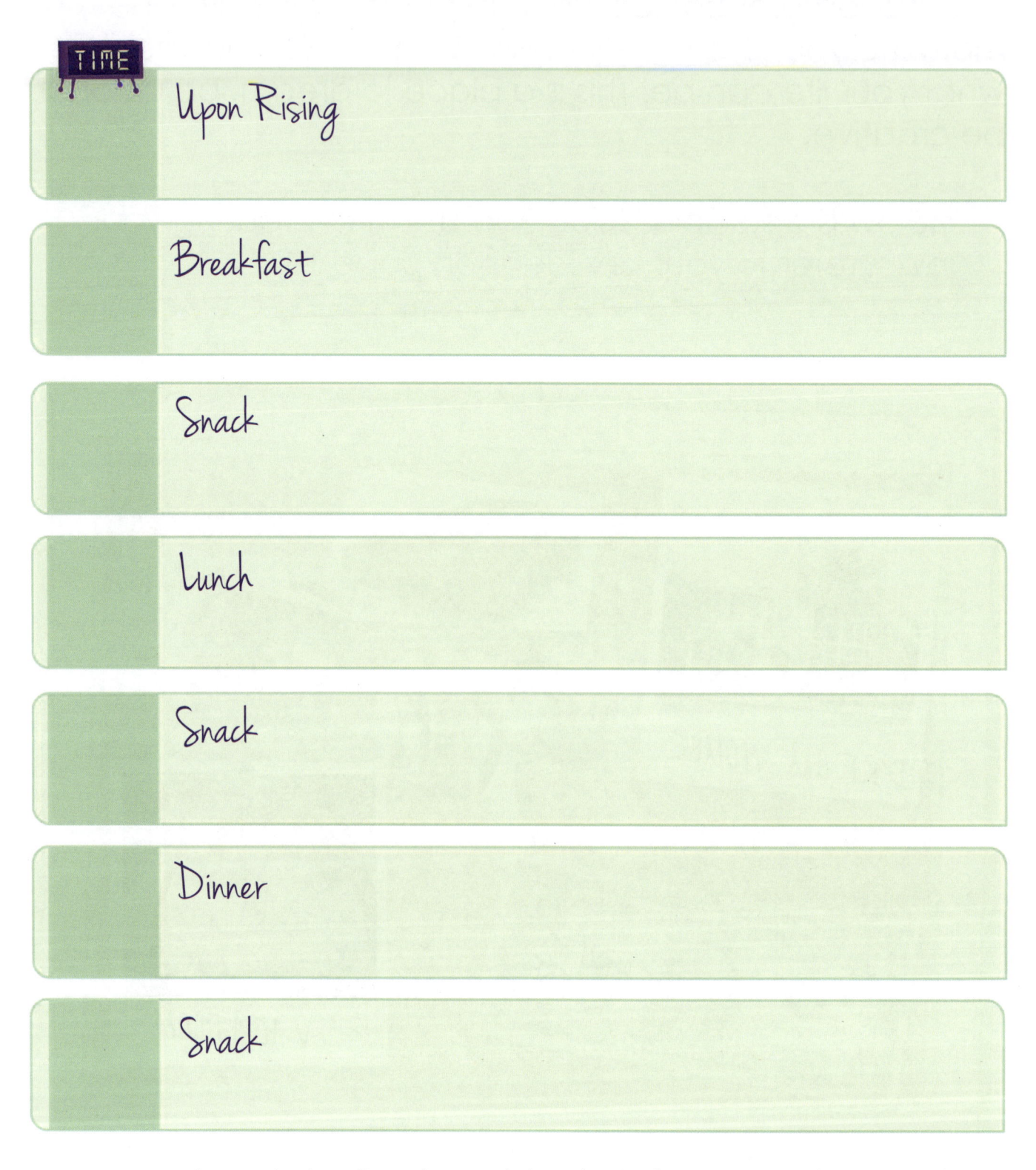

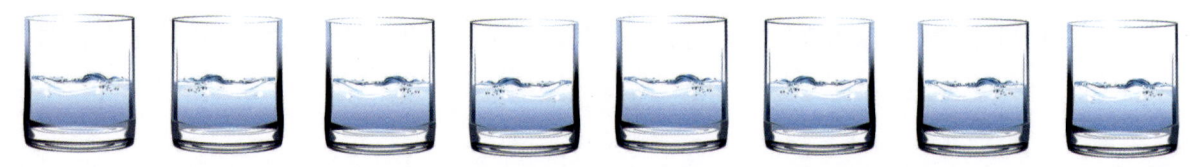

TIME

Upon Rising

Breakfast

Snack

Lunch

Snack

Dinner

Snack

Place a check on the water cups to keep track of every 8oz you drink

Congrats!

You have made it to the end of the 5th week. Time to check in with yourself.

1 How many days this week did you fill in your journal? Write the number, not the excuses.

> Fill in the number of days
> *be honest!*

2 Biggest obstacles this week:
List strategies for overcoming them.

_____
_____
_____
_____
_____
_____

3 What are your goals for the future?

_____
_____
_____
_____
_____
_____

Fun & Healthy e.a.t. Recipe # 5

Cheesecake

> Who says you can't have your cake and eat it too! I grew up in New York eating the best cheesecake... at about 1500 calories per slice! I still love cheesecake but I have found a great way to indulge and not expand my own "bottom line."

Say Cheese to Sugarless Cheesecake

Ingredients

- 2 8oz-packages of cream cheese
- 12 tsp Stevia
- 3 large eggs
- 2 tsp vanilla extract
- 3 cups sour cream
- 1/4 tsp salt
- 3 tbsp fresh lemon juice

Directions

1. Pre-heat oven to 350 degrees F. In a large mixing bowl, beat the cream cheese and Stevia for several minutes until smooth. Add eggs, one at a time and beat each one well into the mixture. Add the lemon juice, vanilla and salt. Blend in the sour cream.

2. Grease an 8-inch springform pan and line the bottom with waxed paper. Make sure to wrap the outside of the pan with heavy-duty tin foil to prevent leakage.

3. Pour the batter into the pan. Set the pan in a large roasting pan surrounded by 1 inch of hot water. Bake for 45 minutes. Turn off the oven without opening the door and let the cake cool for 1 hour.

4. Cover with plastic wrap and refrigerate overnight. Unfold the cake onto a plate the next day and serve with dark chocolate sauce or fresh berries.

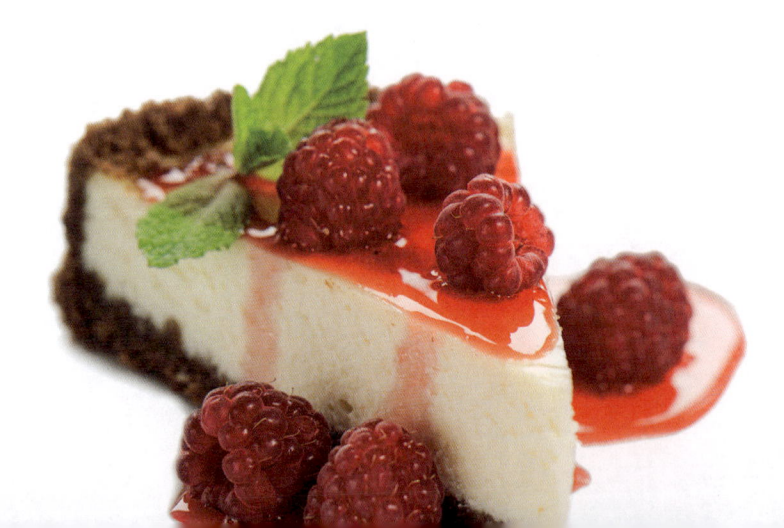

A Message that Counts!

Use clues to decode the quote, said by Buddha, below. Fill in the key as you discover which numbers represent each of the 26 letters of the alphabet.

```
 I                N                 R        S
___   ___ ___ ___ ___ ___   ___   ___ ___ ___
 2     3   9  19   9  21    13     9   9
```

```
___ ___ ___ ___      ___ ___ S
 6  10  24   5        10  24 13
```

```
___ ___ ___ N      ___ ___ N ___      I
 1   9   9  3       17  20 3  9        2
```

```
___ N ___ ___      ___ S ___ ___
 20 3  26  15       3    9   9
```

```
___ ___ ___ ___    R ___ ___ ___ I N S
 6  10  24   5    21 9  11  24 2 3 13
```

```
___ ___      ___ ___     ___ ___ N ___
 5  20        1   9      17  20  3  9
```

— Buddha

Your Key

24	1	4	17	9	7	8	10	2	12	14	26	11
A	B	C	D	E	F	G	H	I	J	K	L	M

3	20	16	18	21	13	5	22	19	6	23	15	25
N	O	P	Q	R	S	T	U	V	W	X	Y	Z

Notes

> Opportunity is missed by most people because its dressed in overalls and looks like work.
>
> - Thomas Edison

Week 6

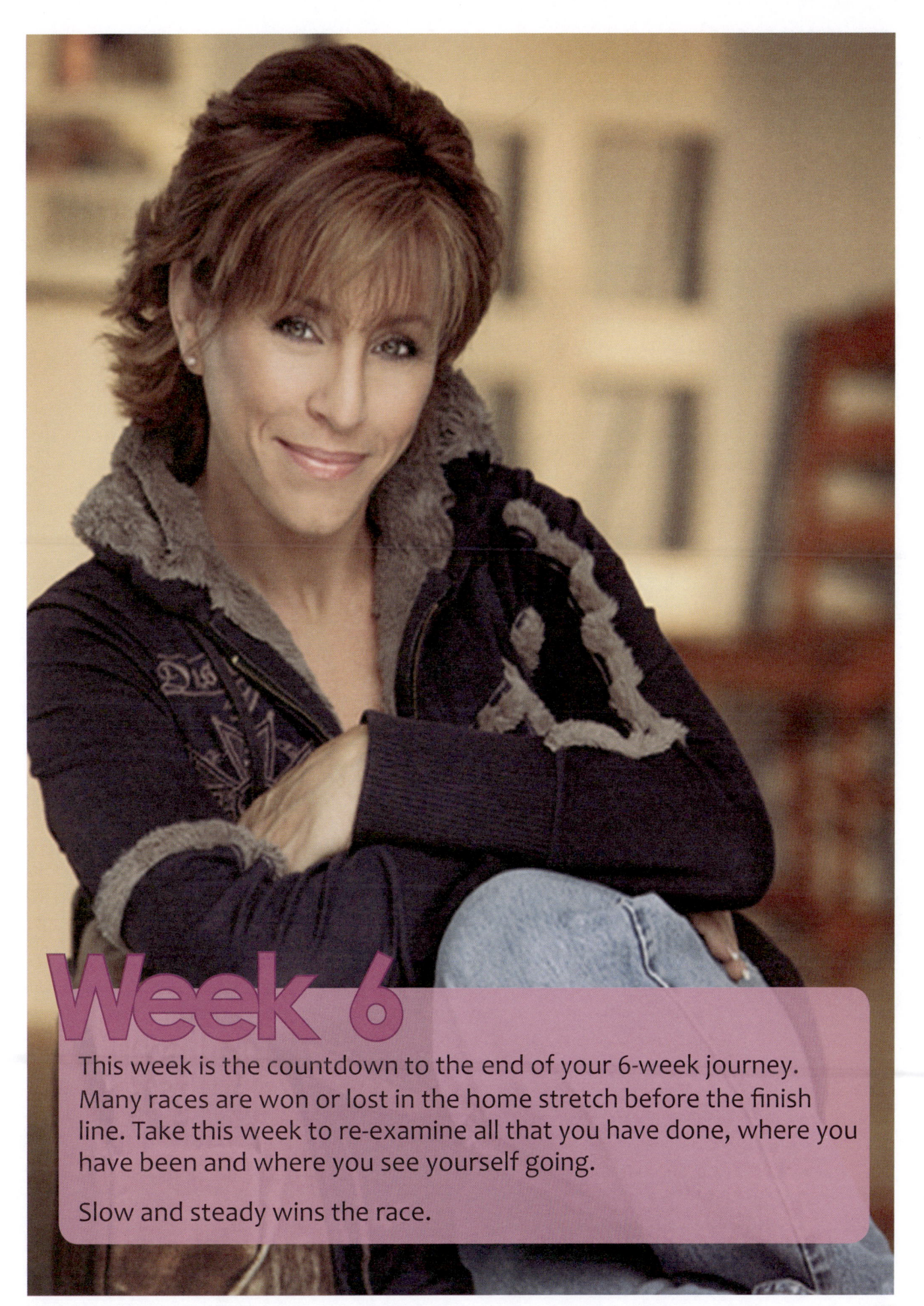

This week is the countdown to the end of your 6-week journey. Many races are won or lost in the home stretch before the finish line. Take this week to re-examine all that you have done, where you have been and where you see yourself going.

Slow and steady wins the race.

What I Eat

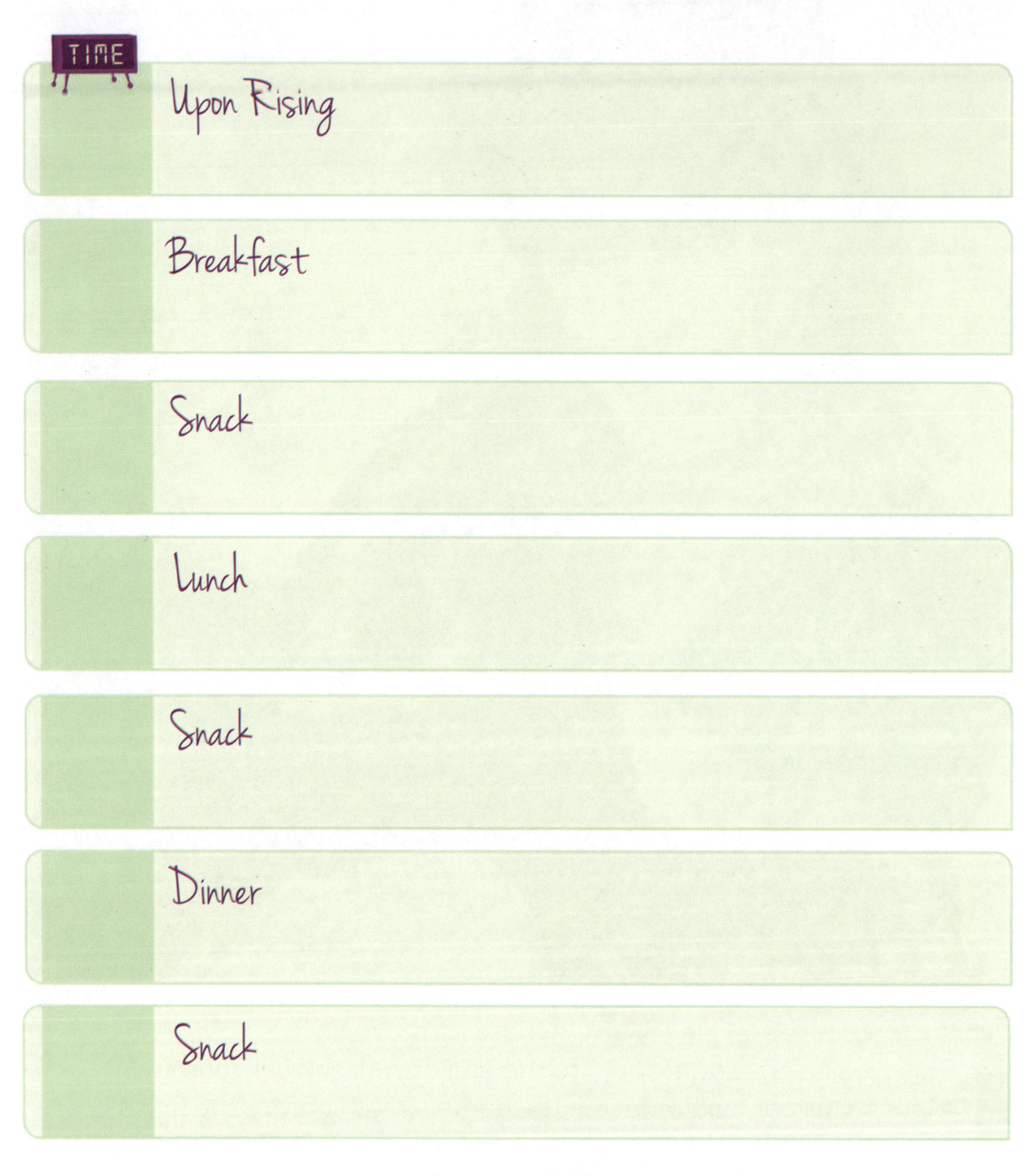

Week 6 — **Day 1**

TIME

- Upon Rising
- Breakfast
- Snack
- Lunch
- Snack
- Dinner
- Snack

Place a check on the water cups to keep track of every 8oz you drink

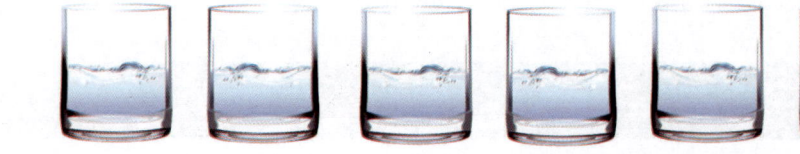

Wisdom (wiz-duhm) noun

1. The quality of being wise.
2. Knowledge of what is true or right coupled with judgement as to action; insight.

As the good witch Glinda said to Dorothy in the Wizard of Oz, *"You've always had the answers inside you – you just have to find them for yourself."* Spend the next few minutes giving yourself some advice that will be wise for you to follow.

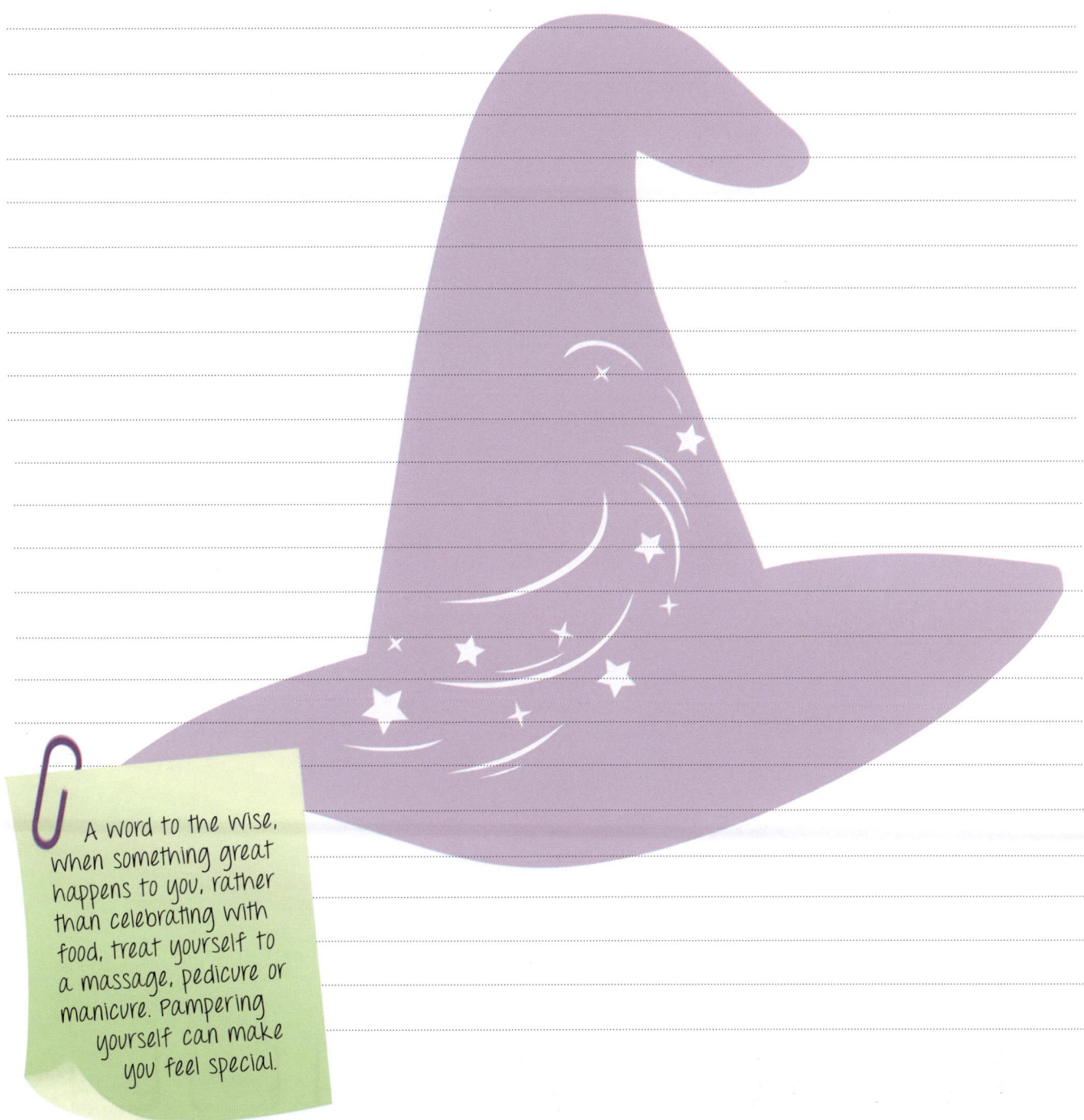

> A word to the wise, when something great happens to you, rather than celebrating with food, treat yourself to a massage, pedicure or manicure. Pampering yourself can make you feel special.

Week 6 — What I Eat — **Day 2**

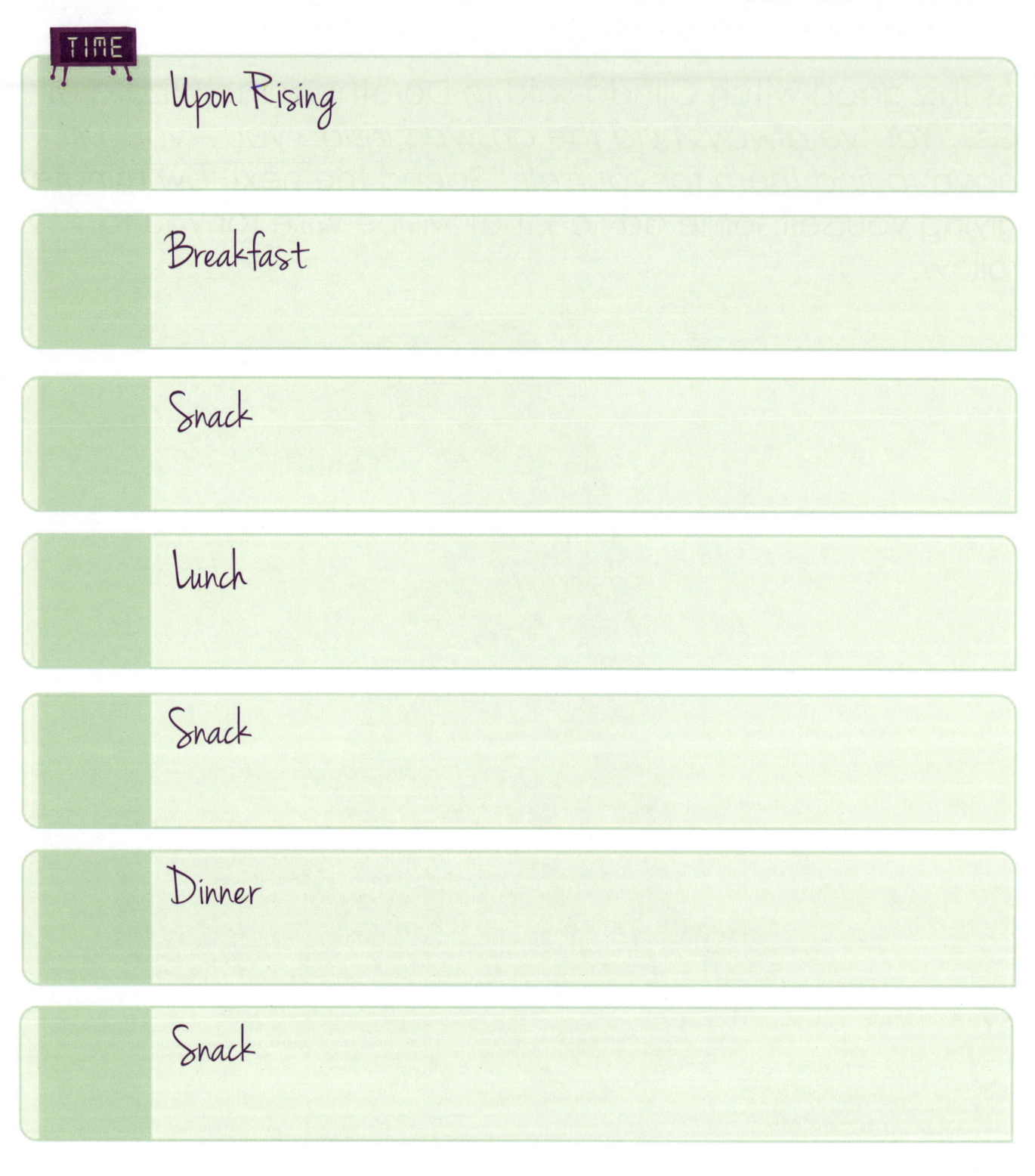

TIME

- Upon Rising
- Breakfast
- Snack
- Lunch
- Snack
- Dinner
- Snack

Place a check on the water cups to keep track of every 8oz you drink

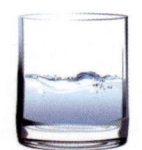

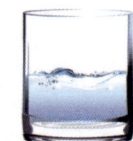

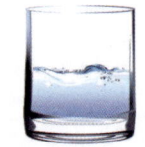

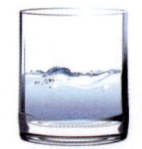

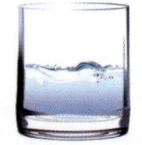

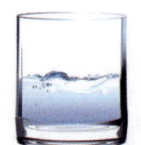

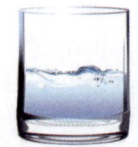

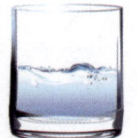

Bad Habits.

Understand and admit to yourself that you have a bad habit. Acknowledging your bad habit is the first step to overcoming it. Ask yourself; what is my bad habit and what is stopping me from getting rid of it?

Got another bad habit you'd like to get rid of?

TIP

Eggs. Scrambled, poached, or hard boiled eggs are a great staple to include in your diet. Eggs are high in sulfur and a wide array of vitamins & minerals. Eat eggs and you may notice healthier hair & nails too.

What I Eat

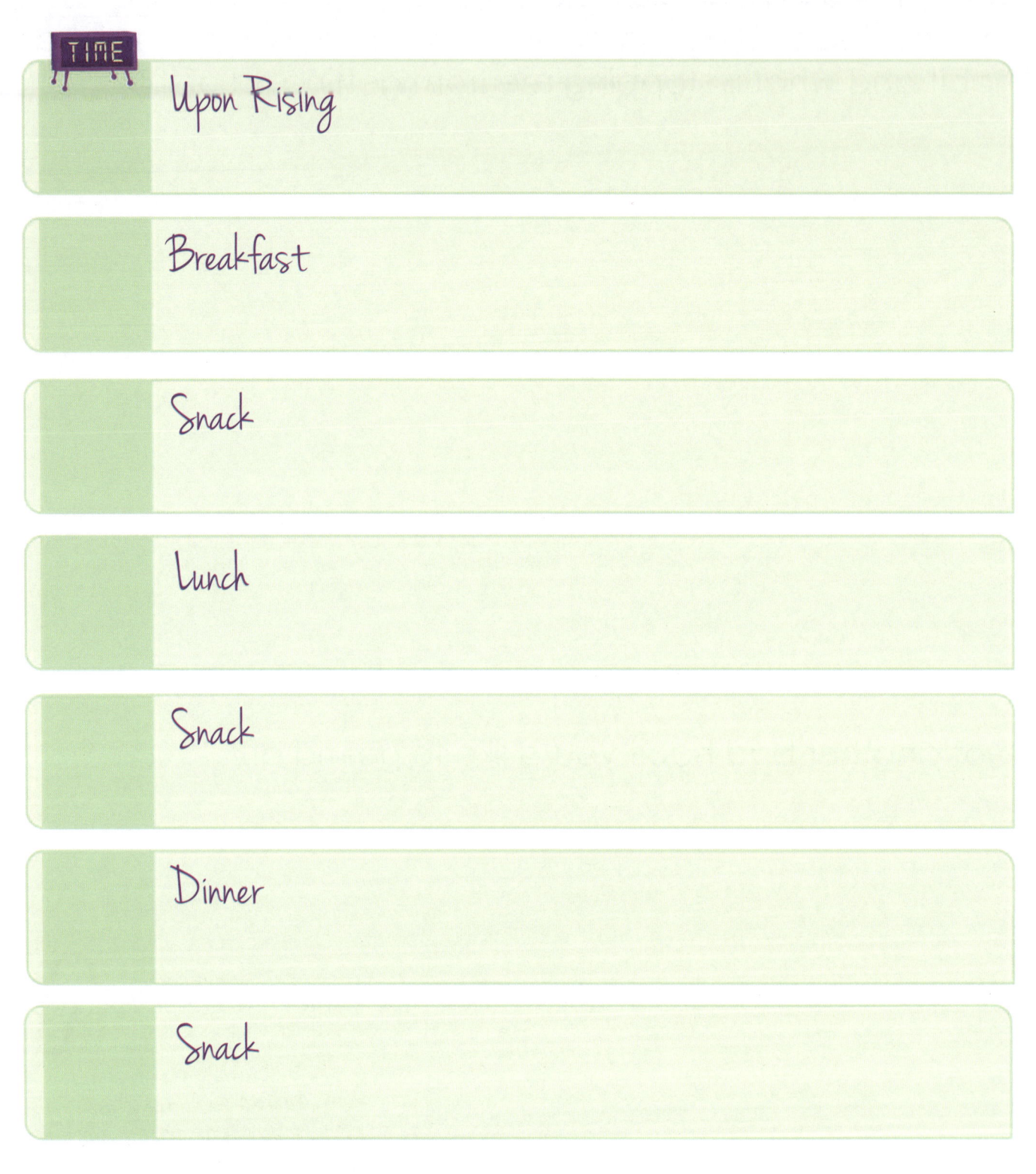

Week 6 — **Day 3**

TIME

- Upon Rising
- Breakfast
- Snack
- Lunch
- Snack
- Dinner
- Snack

Place a check on the water cups to keep track of every 8oz you drink

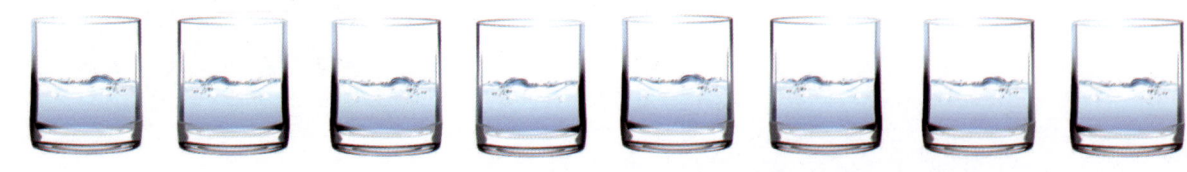

Mend the hems of your life. Try to clean up any emotional messes that may be stopping you from achieving your dreams.

List 3 people whose relationships with you could use a bit of "mending" and why…

1

2

3

> **Tip**
> Try putting down your fork with EVERY bite of your entree. You will eat slower, enjoy the food more and practice finding satisfaction in the art of eating. The science behind eating slower is that it gives your saliva a real chance to start the digestive process.

What I Eat

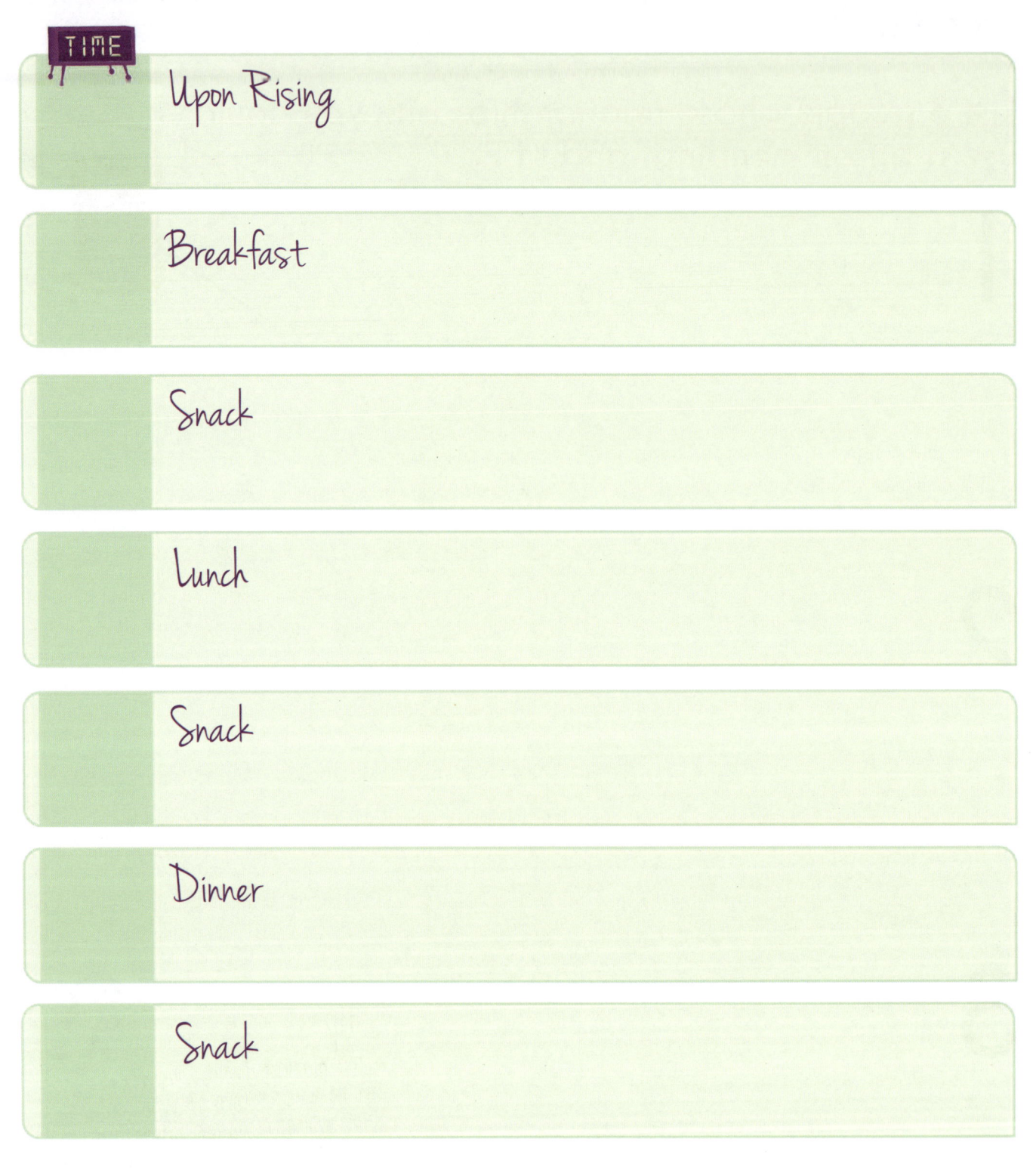

Week 6 — **Day 4**

TIME

- Upon Rising
- Breakfast
- Snack
- Lunch
- Snack
- Dinner
- Snack

Place a check on the water cups to keep track of every 8oz you drink

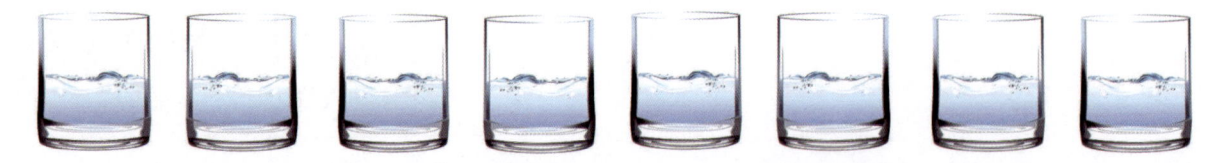

Affirmation

An AFFIRMATION is a declaration that something is true. (whether its actually true at the moment or not)

Create several positive affirmations for yourself. Write them on index cards and place them on your mirror, computer, car dashboard, etc. Examples: I am a talented, worthwhile, creative person. I love my body and appreciate it daily. I can treat myself with compassion and love, I deserve to be happy.

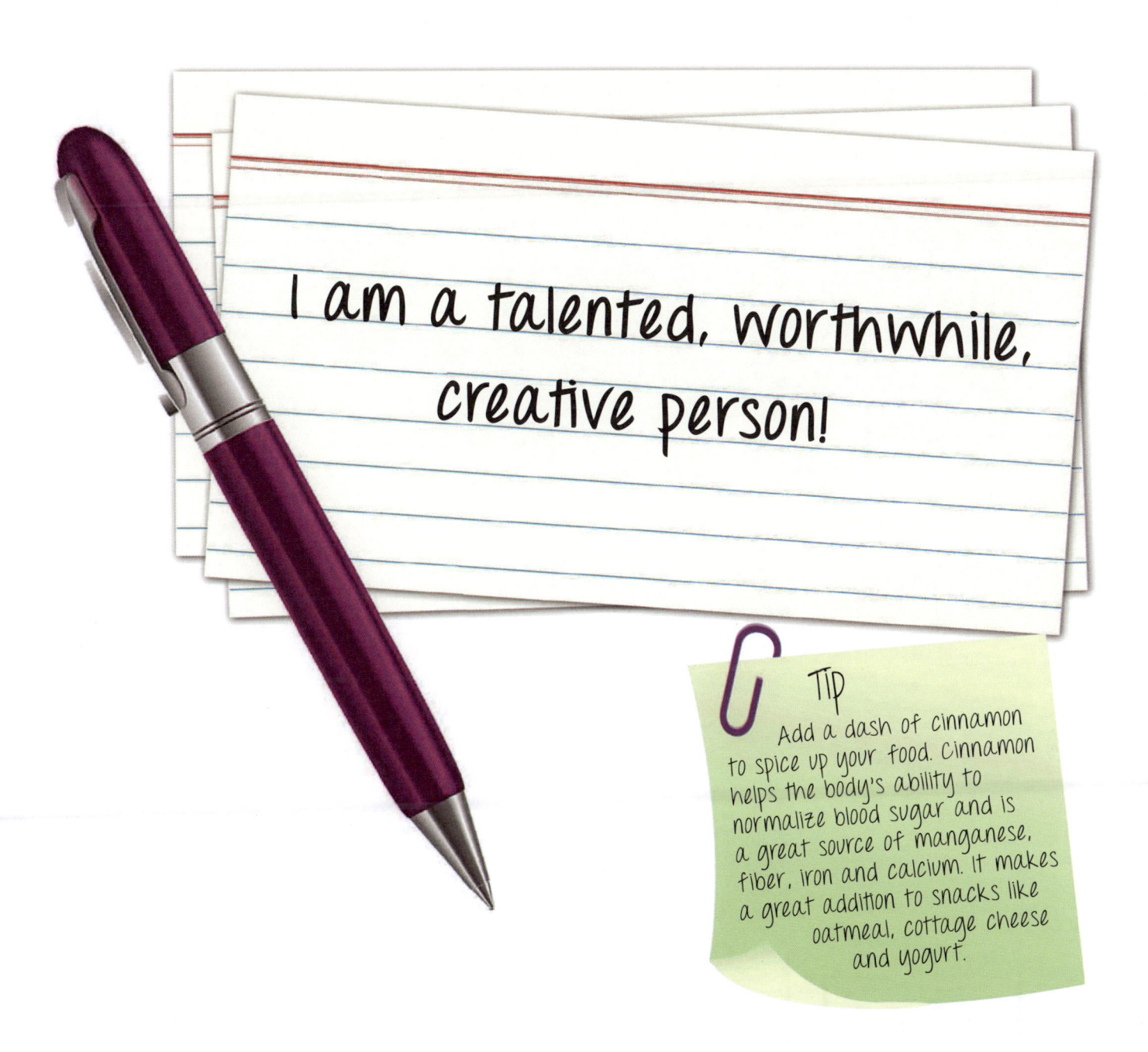

I am a talented, worthwhile, creative person!

TIP
Add a dash of cinnamon to spice up your food. Cinnamon helps the body's ability to normalize blood sugar and is a great source of manganese, fiber, iron and calcium. It makes a great addition to snacks like oatmeal, cottage cheese and yogurt.

What I Eat

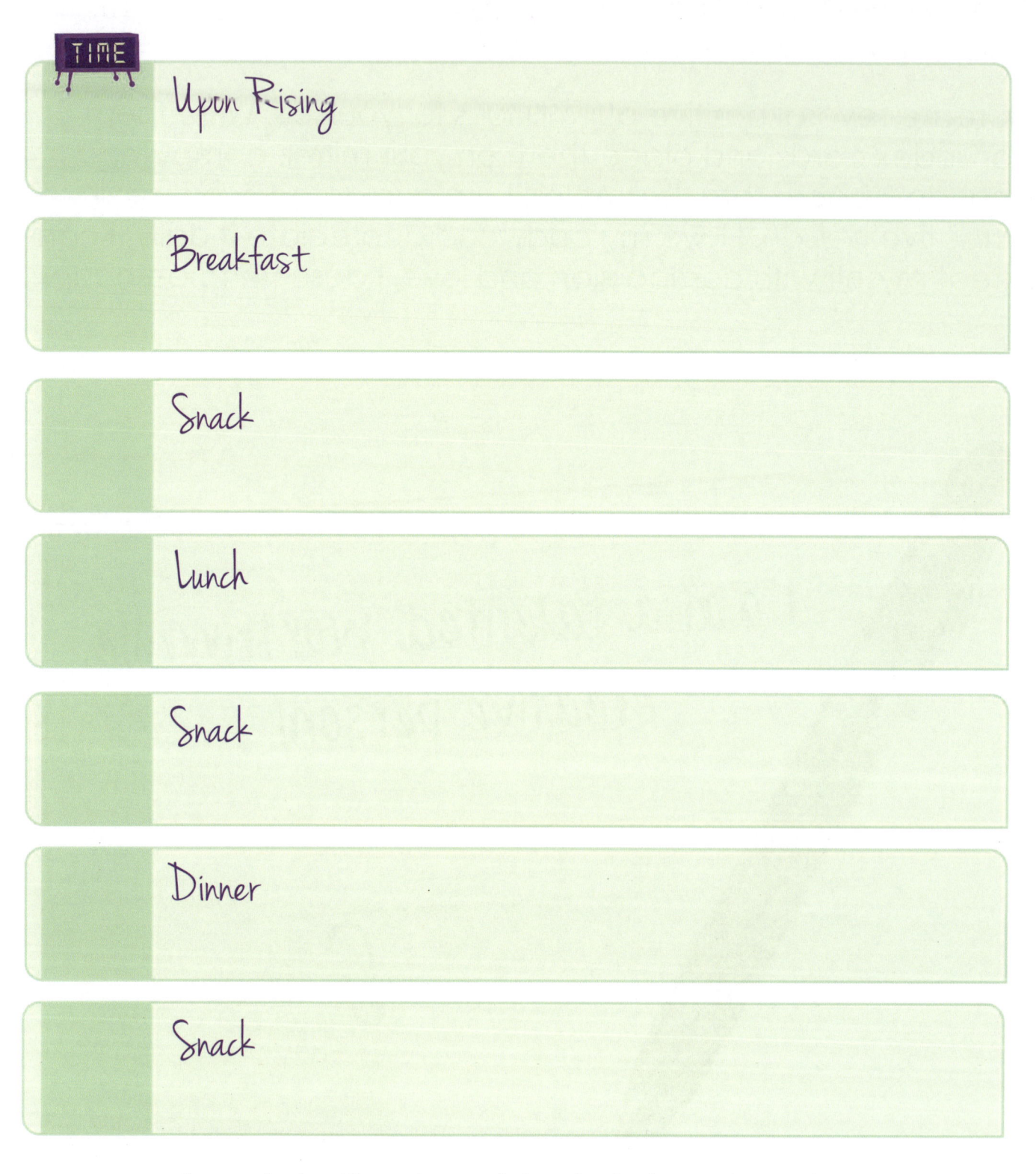

Week 6 — **Day 5**

TIME

- Upon Rising
- Breakfast
- Snack
- Lunch
- Snack
- Dinner
- Snack

Place a check on the water cups to keep track of every 8oz you drink

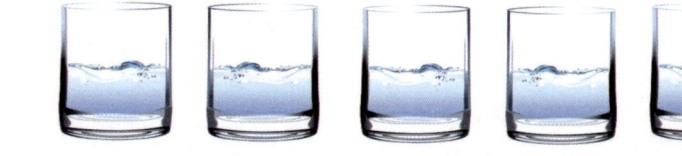

Be prepared for people who may *sabotage* your change. Sabotage may be disguised as cute little children, a loving best friend, or your mate. They may mean well, but be aware of the triggers like, "It's only one dessert," "Everybody cheats, what is wrong with one cookie or chip?" But you can never stop at just one.

List your personal saboteurs.

List your trigger phrases.

What I Eat

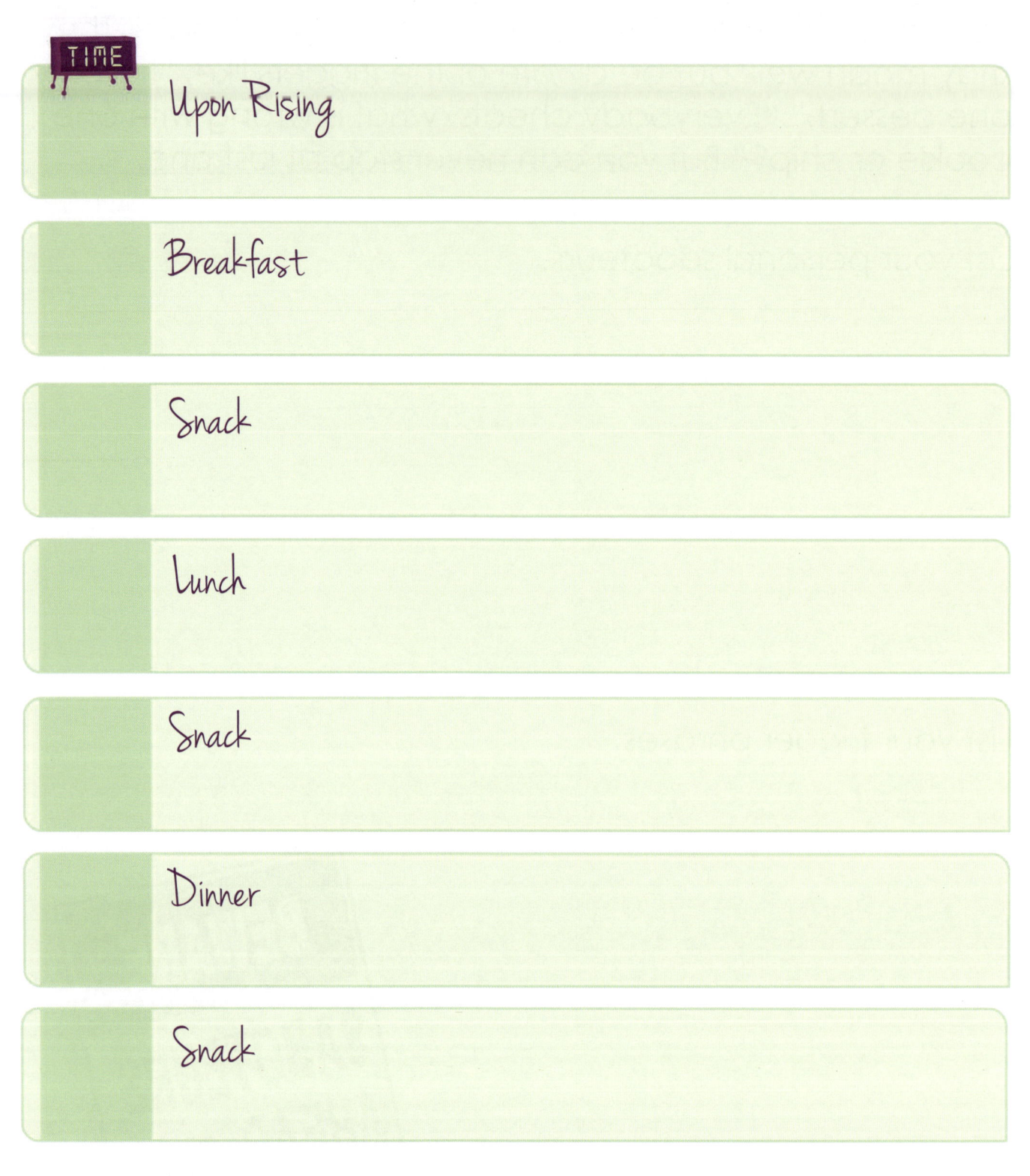

Week 6 — **Day 6**

TIME

- Upon Rising
- Breakfast
- Snack
- Lunch
- Snack
- Dinner
- Snack

Place a check on the water cups to keep track of every 8oz you drink

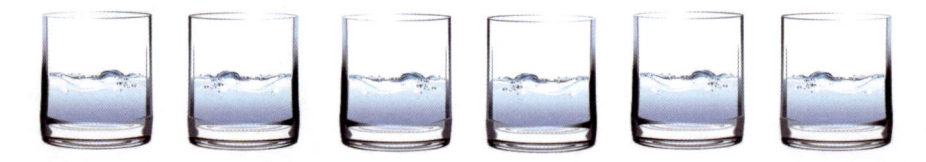

Let's be honest - Really. Write down any fears, anger, or resistance you have at this moment to being successful and enjoying your life - for the rest of your life. Is there any area you are procrastinating in? Write about them.

Any problem well stated is a problem half solved!

TIP

Wine - Some people think wine enhances the enjoyment of food and it does contain resveratrol (an antioxidant) and is high in enzymes. Wine contains 7 calories per gram, so enjoy in moderation.

What I Eat

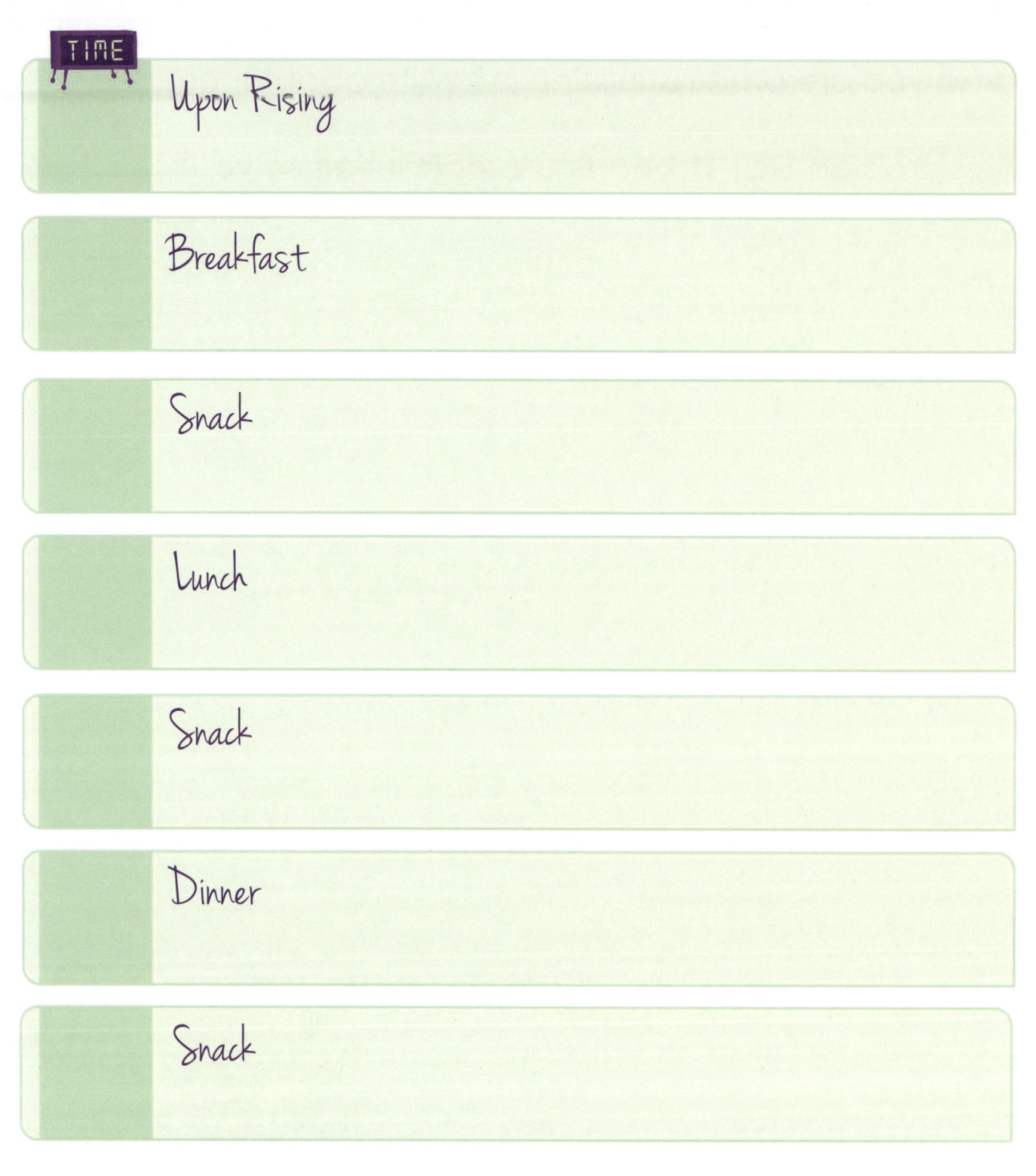

Week 6 — **Day 7**

TIME

- Upon Rising
- Breakfast
- Snack
- Lunch
- Snack
- Dinner
- Snack

Place a check on the water cups to keep track of every 8oz you drink

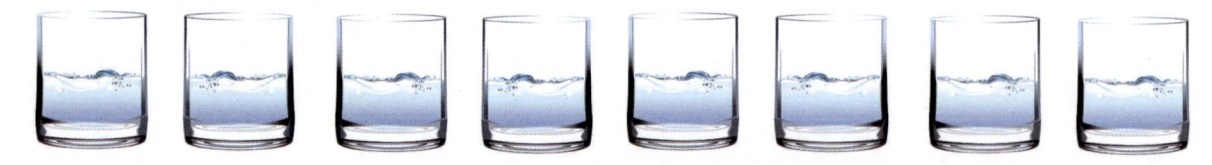

Define Success.

Success comes in many different shapes and sizes. For some, success is owning a big house, or driving a fancy car. For others confined to a wheelchair, success might be getting across the room without anyone's help, or dancing at their child's wedding.

Define what success is for you!

Personal:

Financial:

Success beyond your wildest dreams:

> **TIP**
>
> Try taking yourself on a date. Set aside 2 hours to do something you truly love. A visit to an antique store, a trip to the park, or beach. Perhaps visit the aquarium, art gallery, or the book store.
>
> Nurture yourself.

If you're reading this note, hopefully you have completed this journal, entered in your daily food and wrote a page for each of the exercises. If you haven't, no worries, you did the best you could! ... Or did you?

This journey is all about finding your level of honesty, to check in with yourself in the privacy of your own home and see "who you are", "how you're doing" and "to make positive commitments towards moving forward!"

As the Wicked Witch said to Dorothy in the Wizard of OZ "You've always had the power with you!"

Please take a moment to share some thoughts...

info@myeatjournal.com

My expectation starting my e.a.t. 6 week transformation was...

_____
_____
_____
_____

I was most surprised by....

_____
_____
_____
_____

My commitment moving forward is....

_____
_____
_____
_____

"As a special thank you, this is my gift to e.a.t. READERS."

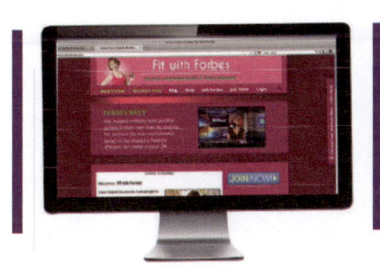

FREE "Fit with Forbes" Membership Offer!

- More than 200 "Member Only" Articles & Videos
- Connect Directly and "Ask Forbes" Questions
- Get Healthy Nutritional Tips
- Videos of Forbes cooking, juicing and "sharing secrets"
- "Member Only" Workout Videos
- Daily motivation to help you achieve your goals!
- Celebrity Interviews and more!

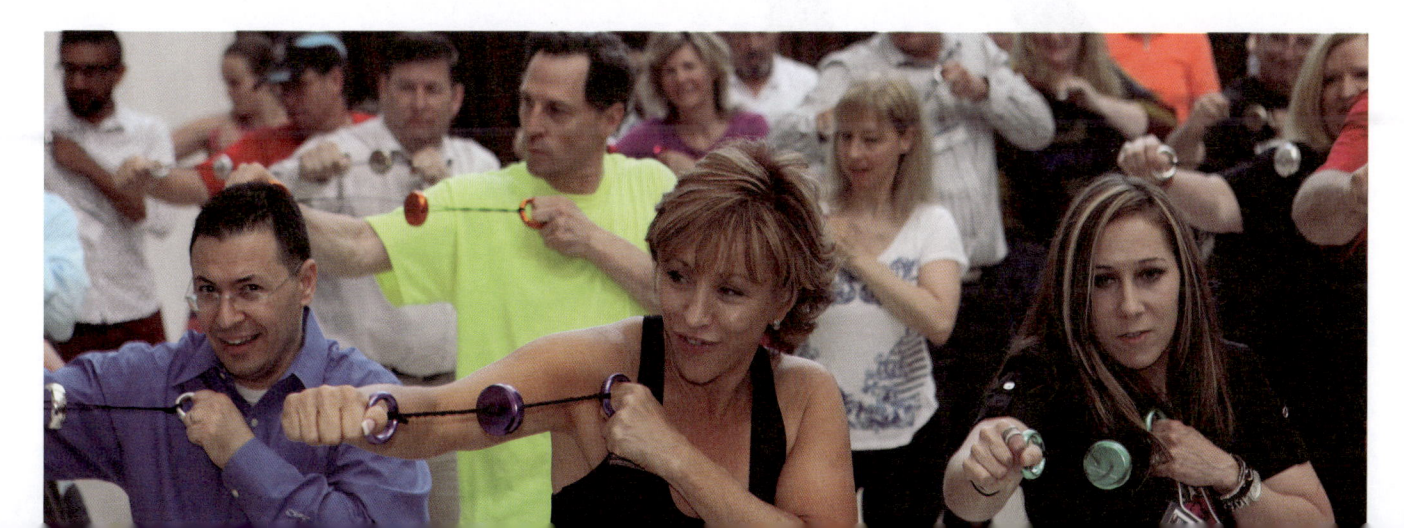

Personal Stats
At the end of your journey

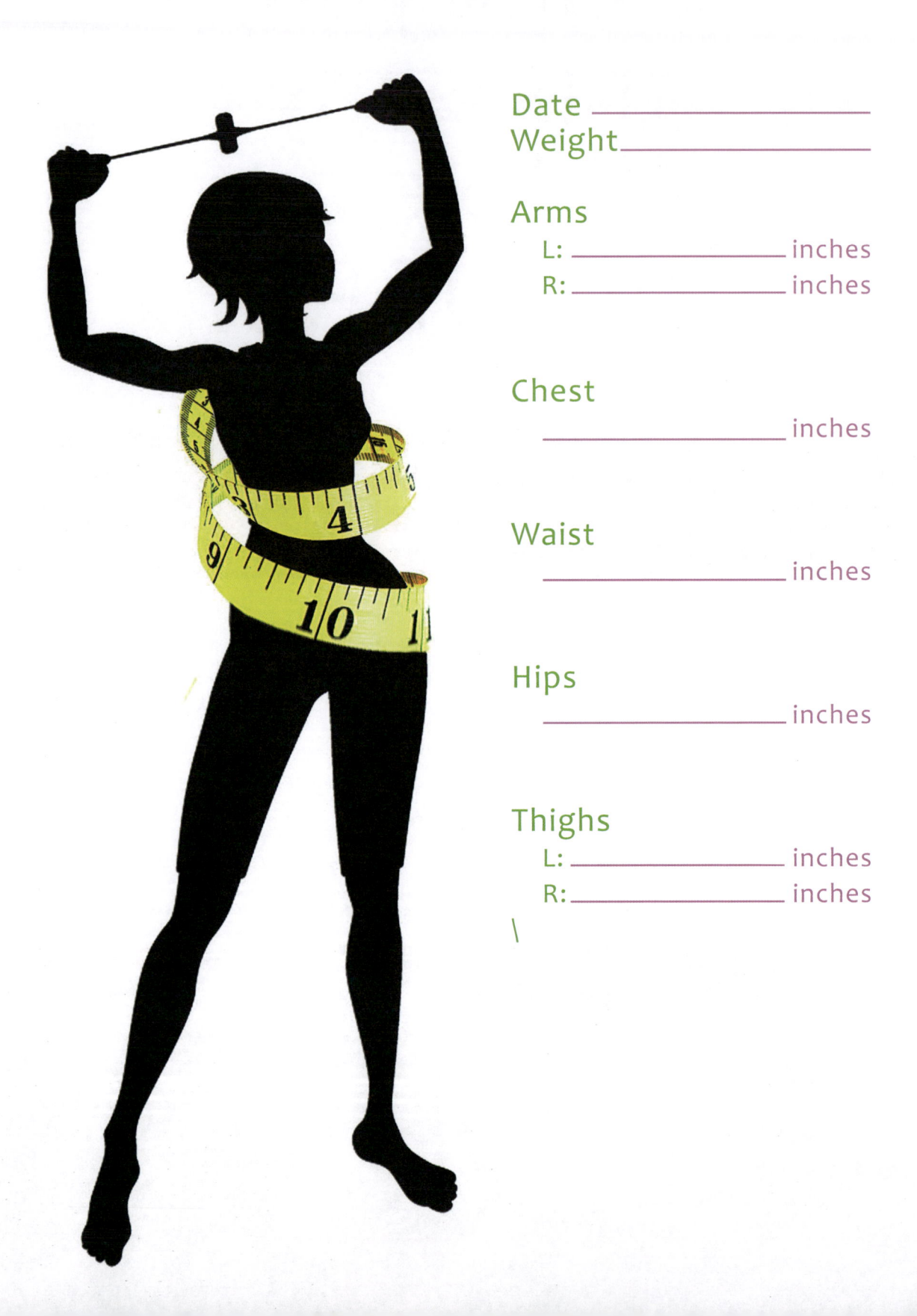

Date _____
Weight _____

Arms
  L: _____ inches
  R: _____ inches

Chest
_____ inches

Waist
_____ inches

Hips
_____ inches

Thighs
  L: _____ inches
  R: _____ inches

Your Success Photo

Congratulations for making it this far! You have completed your goal and you should be proud of what you have accomplished. I would love to hear all about it! Please e-mail your success story along with your before and after photos, to Forbes@MySpinGym.com.

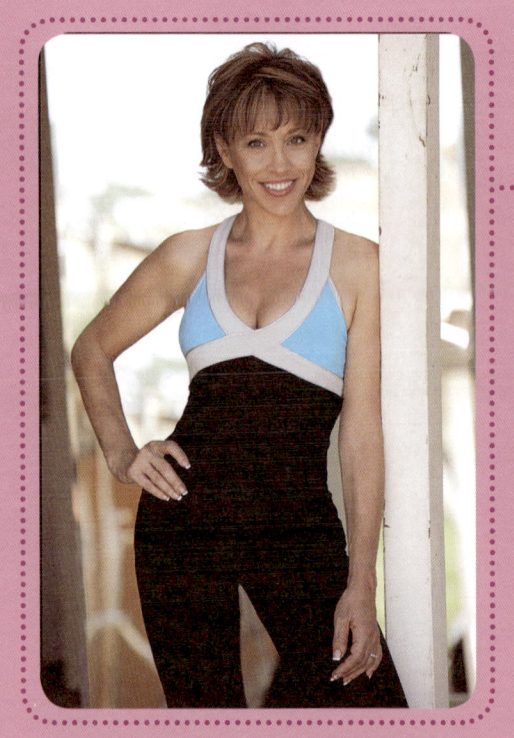

Forbes Riley

Forbes Riley is an award winning national TV host, one of America's leading health & fitness experts, keynote speaker, author and Founder/CEO of the best-selling fitness system: SpinGym. Considered one of the most inspiring people on television, stage and for her coaching, Forbes' unique connection with her audience stems from her own personal journey towards wellness and has helped her create a worldwide brand name in fitness, personal empowerment and business growth and success.

As a motivator and role model, before becoming a media success, Forbes struggled with her own weight, but e.a.t. journaling combined with SpinGym and her unique take on mindset and wellbeing, helped her achieve her personal goals. Now she's dedicated and on mission to help others eliminate the pain and suffering from poor body image, obesity, digestive, issues and mental mindset for overall success and fulfillment.

She began her career as an accomplished actress and dancer in Broadway shows playing opposite the late Christopher Reeve, working with Bob Fosse, and helping to launch The American Dance Machine. Her career spanned to hosting TV shows ESPN (X-Games), TLC (hosting the daily national talk show: "Essentials"), ABC-Family, FIT-TV, and acting in movies/ tv ("24", series lead Fox's "Fashion House", "Picket Fences", "The Practice", "As The World Turns" and more - see IMBD.com for details.).

Forbes' expertise in hosting combined with her passion for health & fitness that lead her to pioneer women in the field of infomercials and on home shopping and being the awarding winning host of two of the most successful infomercials of all time: Power Juicer with legend Jack LaLanne and Montel Williams' Health Master. In 2010, Forbes was recognized as a leader in her field generating more than $2 Billion dollars inducted into the National Fitness Hall of Fame alongside Arnold Schwarzenegger, Joe Weider and Tony Little.

Forbes Riley's crowning jewel in her accomplishments is her media empire headquartered in St. Petersburg, Florida at the Forbes Riley Studios, (a state-of-the-art TV/film production studio and sound stage) and her branded line of fitness solutions and online membership/coaching programs.

And if being an international fitness pioneer isn't enough, Forbes now spends time teaching other entrepreneurs her blueprints for Success. She can be seen live speaking at colleges, corporations, seminars and nationally with her tv talk series, Forbes Living (www.ForbesLivingTV.com).

Contribution and Giving is a gift Forbes received as a young girl when her father suffered a horrific accident and spent 3 years (during high school) in the hospital enduring 15 operations. With an eye towards helping her community and those in need, Forbes is active with a variety of charitable organizations, including Big Brothers/Big Sisters, Veteran WheelChair Games, Clothes to Kids, Dress for Success, SPCA, The Dexter Fund, and many more.

For this inspirational dynamo there is no end in sight as she lives her motto, "Dream It. Believe It. Achieve It." and she's on a mission to empower everyone towards their personal best in all areas of their lives!

For more info, please visit www.ForbesRiley.com and connect on www.Facebook.com/ForbesRileyFANpage.

Acknowledgements

This book encompasses a lifetime of thoughts, struggles, and finally success for me and countless others when it comes to the "battle of the bulge". I only wish this book had been around when I was going through my journey! I'm so happy to be able to share this with you and just know it couldn't have happened without the support of so many wonderful people in my life:

To my Mom and Dad, who raised me with absolute love and the best of intentions, but when it came to food – let's just say it was the 60's and none of us knew better! I miss you both every day, so much, but trust that your spirit is everywhere, continuing to guide me and look after my children. You did such a great job raising me and my sister - my dream is that my children grow to love and honor me as much as I do both of you. To my sister Georgine, you are such a bundle of energy and passion and I have appreciated having you in my life to share all our memories, hopes and dreams.

Thank you Michael Helms - one of the most inspiring photographers I've ever met - It's been a 20 year collaboration that keeps getting better - you always make me look and feel so beautiful - I appreciate your continued belief in me! A picture really is worth a thousand words! And to Perry Gallagher, another genius photographer who pushes me to dig inside and find the truth in all the photos he takes. The images that both of you shot for this book help make it so unique and special.

To my friend and mentor, the Godfather of Fitness, Jack LaLanne - your words live on in me and my children. "If man made it, don't eat it". You changed my life and thanks to you and your amazing wife, Elaine, I am working to continue your legacy of eating good food and daily exercise.

Patricia Bragg, you are a ray of sunshine and I think of you EVERY morning as I drink Bragg's Apple Cider Vinegar, comforted by the fact that celebrities from Katy Perry to Clint Eastwood share in my morning ritual.

My friends and advisors, far too many to list in this book, I thank you. Success is rarely achieved alone and I am humbled by the brilliant nurturing souls that have influenced my life. You have witnessed my struggles and always stood by me - this is the good part where we get to celebrate. I pray that anyone who suffers with an eating problem, struggles with their weight or feels "less than" because of their compulsions, finds relief, peace of mind and sanity so they can enjoy their lives and grow to their full potential.

To Dennis Mancuso, who initially helped guide my vision from thought to computer. Tom and Barbara Hale, who raised such a caring and talented daughter, Jaki, who joined me on a journey that neither of us had planned. Jaki, your talent and thinking outside of the box will serve you well in your career and life; I am happy to have been there at the beginning.

A group hug to my advisors who graciously answered my phone calls, texts, and emails no matter what the time of day or night and motivated me just by being amazing people - Joe Theismann, John Baudhin, Karen Glubis, Patricia Stockhausen, Mike Emmerman, Andi Matheny, Kathy Kaehler, John Abdo, Briana Michel, and Tony Little. I know there are many more wonderful people to thank—so please don't be upset if I failed to mention your name specifically.

To my dear Frances Diaz, gone but not forgotten. Your commitment and infectious laugh made an indelible impact on me and my family. I hear you in my dreams cheering me on!

To my supportive HSN team from Mindy Grossman to Jane Dyer, Joanna Schottler and Carrie Koch – I want to thank you for your continued faith in the Forbes Riley brand. You fueled the fire of SpinGym and have helped me live the dream of helping others get fit, happy and healthy - so grateful to you all - you work so tirelessly to make us look good!

And finally to my family - you share me with the world, let me go and do "my work thing" and still think I'm a great mom -- that means so much to me. Ryker and Makenna, your curiosity, unconditional love and energy inspire me every day. To Tom, what a rollercoaster! I'm grateful that you've held on for the wild ride. Your support, generosity and the best homecooked meals ever have made this a journey worth sharing. I have never known someone who cares so much and works so hard. And there's more people who've touched my heart and made this possible, you know who you are.

Thank you.

Notes

Forbes Fit and Fun Answers

Below find the answers to your weekly puzzles throughout your journey!

Crossword Puzzle (page 35)

Across
7 Protein
8 Halloween
10 Femur
11 Dumbbells
14 Water
15 Detox
16 Heat
18 Grains
19 You
20 SpinGym

Down
1 Carbohydrate
2 Fonda
3 Functions
4 Pilates
5 Jack LaLanne
6 Health
9 Bikram
12 Sodium
13 Nutrition
17 Turkey

Missing Letter (page 93)

Artichokes
beets
mangoes
plums
Lettuce
Cherries
Papayas
Cabbage
zucchini
lemons
kiwi
broccoli
watermelon
squash

Healthy Choices

Wordsearch (page 55)

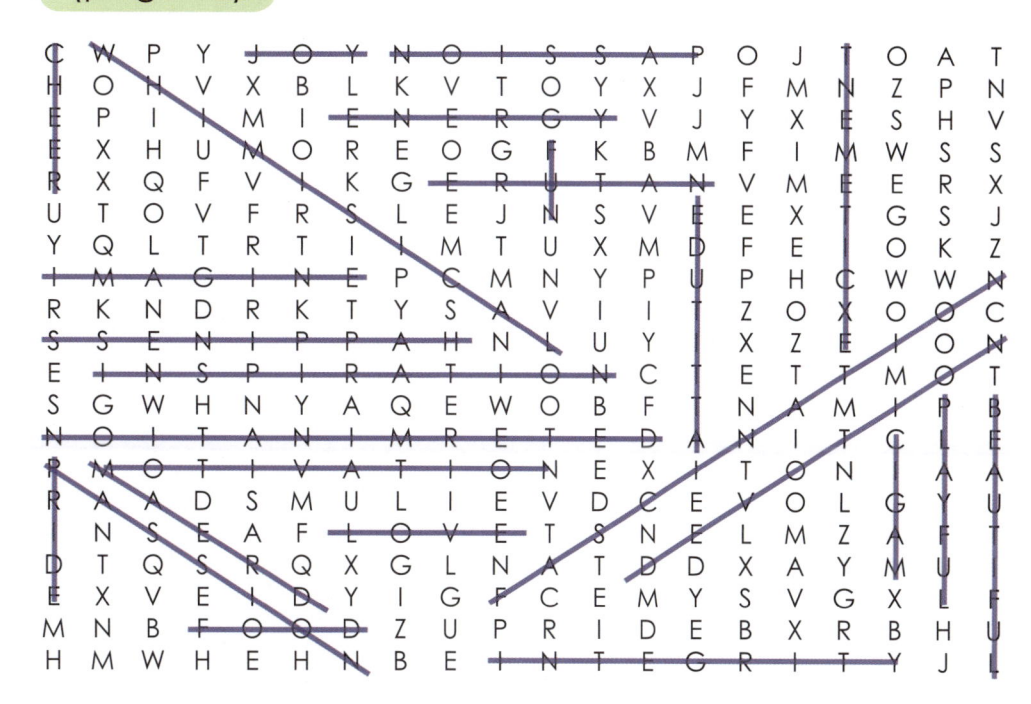

Health Jumble (page 75)

vegetable
fitness
workouts
asparagus
lemons
chicken
steak
cauliflower
lettuce
swordfish
attitude

journal
success
inspiration
physical
strong
cholesterol
vitamins
organic
natural
healthier
water

A Message that Counts! (page 111)

I Never See What Has Been Done, I Only See What Remains to be done.

- *Buddha*

135

Notes